PowerFoods

Power
Foods

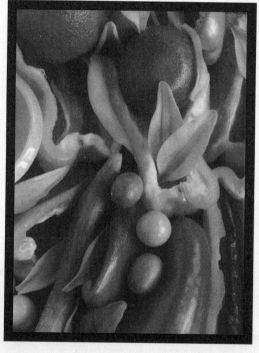

**GOOD FOOD, GOOD HEALTH WITH
PHYTOCHEMICALS, NATURE'S OWN ENERGY BOOSTERS**

*Featuring 140 Delicious Recipes by Executive Chefs
Barry Correia and Carl DeLuce*

Stephanie Beling, M.D.

HarperPerennial
A Division of HarperCollinsPublishers

First HarperPerennial edition published 1998.

Designed by Stephanie Tevonian
Photography by Karen Capucilli

The Library of Congress has catalogued the hardcover edition as follows:

Beling, Stephanie.
    Powerfoods : good food, good health with phytochemicals, nature's own energy boosters / by Stephanie Beling. — 1st ed.
      p. cm.
    Includes bibliographical references and index.
    ISBN 0-06-017454-4
    1. Nutrition.   2. Botanical chemistry.   3. Vegetables—Composition.   I. Title.
RA784.B367   1997
613.2—DC21   97-1046

ISBN 0-06-092954-5 (pbk.)

99 00 01 02 ❖/RRD 10 9 8 7 6 5 4 3 2

Contents

Contents

Acknowledgments

*t*his book would not exist if it were not for the faith, support, and expertise of a group of people it has been my privilege to know. It's a pleasure to be able to thank them here.

First, my editors. For her enthusiastic embrace of the idea of a book on PowerFoods, I am indebted above all to Susan Friedland, Director of Cookbook Publishing at HarperCollins. Jennifer Griffin, with her meticulous attention to detail, was invaluable in helping me pull the manuscript together and point it in the right direction. And Megan Newman has been both indispensable and a delight in bringing the book to final fruition.

To executive chefs Barry Correia and Carl DeLuce, my thanks for their appreciation of the power of PowerFoods and for their mouthwatering recipes. Janice Thomas's typing skills were an object lesson in creating order out of chaos, and Susanna Margolis provided considerable editorial assistance—and fun discussions. My thanks to them both.

Most of all, I want to acknowledge my colleagues at Canyon Ranch in the Berkshires, two expert nutritionists—Kathie Swift, M.S., R.D., Director of Nutrition, and Rebecca Bouchard, R.D.—for their extraordinarily helpful comments, suggestions, and creatively stimulating discussions.

On the most deeply personal level, thanks of course to my husband, Carl Beling, for being a dependable source of strength and calm at all times, and to my daughter Kate Squires for sharing her remarkable gifts of comprehension and communication.

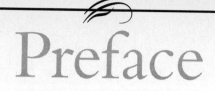

Preface

*t*his book is about ten food groups that are particularly beneficial against the afflictions of our time—cancer and cardiovascular disease, obesity and hypertension, the low energy and chronic illness that plague our society. Quite simply, these PowerFoods contain hidden properties, called phytochemicals, that can help prevent these afflictions, retard the aging process, and improve and enhance our ability to enjoy life. My aim in writing the book is twofold: to issue a call to action and to sing a paean to the pleasures of eating.

Take Action

The action I hope you will take—and this book offers help for getting started—is once and for all to take control of your diet and commit to healthy eating for a lifetime. The incentives are great—feeling and looking better; a greatly lowered risk of disease; and a slowing of the aging process.

We Literally Are What We Eat

It is no cliché to say that we are what we eat. Rather, it is scientific fact. The food we eat becomes us. Through the physiological processes of digestion, absorption, and metabolism, our bodies convert food into muscle, liver, blood and bone. That apple, sweet potato, and garden fresh salad—or that doughnut, fried chicken and bag of potato chips is destined to become our heart, brain, or lungs. Nothing except the air we breathe and the water we drink, is as essential to our bodies' existence as food. It is the bedrock of health.

And good food is the bedrock of good health. The better we eat, the stronger our bones, the more flexible our muscles, the more efficient our liver, heart, and brain.

When I began studying medicine, these facts, although known, played little role in the curriculum. Medicine, at that time was strictly allopathic; the emphasis was on elaborate diagnostic tools, pharmaceuticals, surgery and high-technology scientific advances. There was not a word about the role of nutrition in the prevention or treatment of disease.

Today, for the first time, the number of obese people exceeds the number of appropriate-weight people in all age groups-but especially among women aged 40 to 64. At one time or another, almost everyone has been on a diet, yet the vast majority of dieters are today fatter than before their diet.

But obesity is not the only problem. Our "advanced" civilization has also produced such phenomena as pollution and overcrowding, while the fast pace of our lives has produced a number of stresses and strains. Not surprisingly, the incidence of such diseases as hypertension and Type II diabetes is up. At the same time, people's level of energy and sense of calm are down. As a physician, I am regularly called upon to treat the results of this fast-paced lifestyle.

Since graduating from medical school, my most important teachers have been my patients. In so many of the individuals I treat for obesity, hypertension, diabetes, and high cholesterol levels, the clear cause has been too many calories with too little nutrition. Drugs and surgery are not just inadequate against these ailments, they have very often proven inappropriate. Instead, I have added to my medical black bag such therapies as changing patients' eating habits, increasing their activity, and encouraging stress management.

At the same time, medical research has been confirming what observation has suggested. The science of nutrition has increasingly demonstrated that eating habits, lifestyle, and behavior are the cause of many of the ailments of our time. It's official: by changing eating habits, lifestyle, and behavior, we can prevent and treat these ailments, and we can gain the benefits of energy, fitness, and long-term well-being.

The Pleasures of Eating

The PowerFoods themselves, also demonstrate how extraordinary is Nature's bounty—in the variety of tastes and textures, in the palette of their colors, striking enough to make a rainbow look pale by comparison. These have been the basic, natural foods of mankind for eons-widely available, easy to prepare, enticing to look at, delicious to eat. The pleasures of eating healthfully are the pleasures of eating well; they are pleasures to be savored and enjoyed.

"PowerFoods" includes a hundred and forty recipes covering everything from a fancy dinner party to a picnic lunch, from a summer barbecue to a cold-weather soup, from cocktails for thirty to brunch for two. In addition, throughout the book, you'll find suggestions, anecdotes, hints meant to trigger your own imagination. For imagination is the one essential ingredients you must bring to healthy eating.

My own interest in healthy food extends right into the garden. One of the great joys in my life is to plant tiny seeds into the rich brown-black earth, nourish them with compost, then watch the seeds transform into a multicolored landscape of vegetables and fruits. Each year, it is a miracle to me all over again.

But come late August, when the harvest is upon us and the bushel baskets overflow, that is when imagination is called for. What to do with all this produce coming in at once—broccoli, carrots, potatoes, zucchini, cabbage, cucumbers, onions, and more—especially when you have a job, manage a household, and decide to write a book. My solution is Harvest Vegetable Soup, to be enjoyed all year round. Nothing could be easier:

Wash and cut into chunks—do not peel!—various amounts of the above vegetables and/or any others that might be around. Toss everything into your largest pot, then add vegetable stock about three-fourths of the way up. I use vegetable bouillon cubes or a pack or two of dried vegetable soup and water. Season with whatever appeals to you at the moment, and always use garlic. Last summer, my favorite seasoning included caraway seeds, two or three cloves, a pinch of ginger, a sprinkling of fresh thyme and sage, (or parsley and dill) and salt and pepper to taste—but this will probably give way to a new concoction next summer. Bring all the ingredients in the pot to a boil, cover, then simmer for several hours until the vegetables can be mashed with a fork. Coarsely puree in portions in a blender and put into freezer containers. What a convenience it is, when company suddenly appears, to defrost and heat enough for lunch or dinner. And what a treat it is on a brisk autumn day to come home to this welcome taste of summer after a nice walk in the woods surrounding our home.

Above all, what a sense of well-being there is in the very taste of this PowerFood soup—a cocktail of nutritive and phytochemical compounds that remain unprocessed, their power undimmed, as they move directly from their natural state to your soup bowl. It is the taste of good health. Nothing could be more delicious.

Richmond, Massachusetts
June 1997

Preface

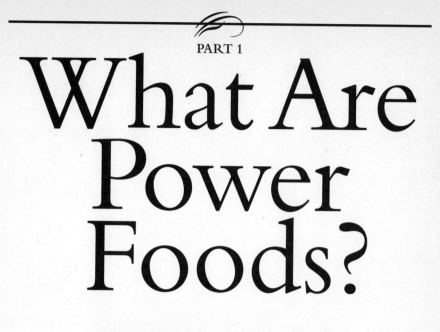

PART 1

What Are Power Foods?

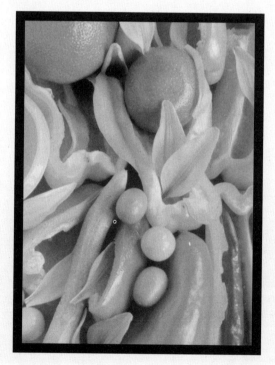

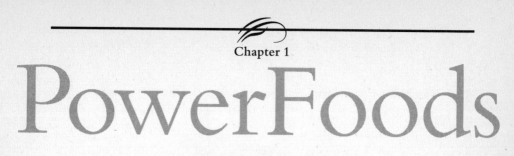

Chapter 1

PowerFoods

WHAT THEY ARE, WHY WE NEED THEM

The doctor of the future will give no medicine, but will interest his patients in the care of the human frame, in diet, and in the cause and prevention of disease.
—THOMAS A. EDISON

Let food be your medicine.
—HIPPOCRATES

*C*all it the American paradox: the United States, one of the richest and most powerful nations in history, is entering the twenty-first century in poor health and in weak physical condition. It needn't be so; it doesn't have to be so. Eating right is one way to correct the paradox. Making the ten food groups I call PowerFoods the center of your diet is a great way to eat right, to actually prevent disease and boost health through diet.

Ironies abound in the American paradox. We have so many opportunities to be healthy. Advances in science and technology have brought the practice of medicine to an unprecedented level of achievement. Today, we can recover from diseases and accidents that would have been fatal at any other time in human history. We work out in gyms and health clubs whose numbers multiply. We can go to spas, take wellness vacations, enjoy eco-holidays. The Information Age assaults us with data about health and fitness. We can satisfy our curiosity about the latest health advice or nutritional news by calling up, reading up, tuning in, or logging on.

Yet in the face of these opportunities, Americans suffer chronic degenerative diseases to an extent that is unique in history and beyond the incidence of such diseases in other, less developed countries. We are gravely ill to the tune of 1.2 million cancer diagnoses a year, four million individuals disabled from arthritis, some 16 million ill with diabetes—even if about half of them do not know it. Every thirty-three seconds in this country, someone dies from heart disease. One in three adult Americans—and one in five American children—is overweight. Overfed but undernourished, 61 million Americans fall within the scientific definition of obesity. We don't like the way we look, and we don't like the way we feel.

We seek help in prescriptions for antidepressants, antihypertensives, antibiotics—and in nonprescription remedies marketed and sold with the promise of relieving tension, reducing weight, lowering blood pressure, boosting energy. Eighty million times a year, an American goes on a diet. Nearly a third of women between the ages of nineteen and thirty diet at least once a month.

Afraid of disease, persuaded by the images of popular culture to fear old age, our response is to put our hope in the search for a magic potion—a single substance that will not just sustain life, not just enhance health and fitness, but actually stave off or even cure the dreaded diseases of our age—cancer, heart disease, infections, arthritis, diabetes, gastrointestinal illness, not to mention such "sicknesses" of our society as obesity, hypertension, depression, mental illness, and more. This search for a single "magic bullet" explains the success of powder-drink meals and vitamin supplements. But there is no such thing as an Elixir of Life. There never was. Chances are there never will be.

Instead of sorcery, we must look to science. Instead of fantasizing about a miracle capsule that will make us healthy and fit, we must concentrate on what is within our control. What we eat, how much, and how often is certainly within our control, and it has a tremendous impact on our health. Eating PowerFoods on a regular basis can have the most beneficial impact on our health, can make us feel good, look good, and live longer. This book shows you how to make PowerFoods a part of your diet for a healthier, happier life.

The Relationship Between Health and Diet

Of all the variables of modern life, diet is one that each individual can directly and entirely control. Research in and out of the laboratory is confirming an old truth: We are what we eat, and if there is a magic bullet for health, its trajectory goes right through mealtime.

The scientific community is virtually unanimous that changes in diet can improve a person's health and help prevent the chronic diseases and degenerative conditions that plague us. In fact, it is estimated that seven out of the top ten causes of death can be positively affected by an improved diet. Despite all the evidence, however, we seem reluctant to do what science and medicine recommend.

Americans have been assured time and again that they will be healthier and will feel better if they shift the proportions in the typical American diet of meat-first-vegetables-last. Four major reports on diet and health published in the last several years recommended reducing the consumption of dietary fat and increasing the consumption of complex carbohydrates and fiber. The 1990 Dietary Guidelines for Americans specifically recommended a low-fat diet with plenty of vegetables, fruits, and grain products. When the Department of Agriculture modified its Food Guide Pyramid in 1993, based on recommendations from a joint Harvard–World Health Organization study, it made the base of the pyramid a combination of grains, fruits, vegetables, and legumes. The Food and Drug Administration recommends five servings a day of fruit and vegetables. Any doctor will tell you that you are better off when cheeseburgers and chocolate yield to carrots and cantaloupe.

Every time another headline proclaims that certain foods offer health benefits or that certain other foods threaten ill effects, people react—at least, in the short term. They give up red meat, fill up on fiber, and start popping pills containing the synthetic version of the latest "health" food. Such responses are just variations on the search for a magic potion, and the results are typically just as disappointing:

First, diets based on deprivation tend to collapse after a short time.

After the deprivation comes the binge eating. When you treat yourself to a huge steak as a reward for months of no red meat, the result can be a serious jolt to the system. As for weight loss, 95 percent of dieters have regained the weight they've lost, and then some, in five years. In fact, studies show that most short-term weight-loss diets are just as unhealthy as the bad eating habits they try to correct. There is more, not less, obesity in the country; we have more, not fewer, problems with our immune systems; and we certainly have not won the war against disease. The bottom line: Deprivation simply does not work.

Second, forcing yourself to eat one kind of food in particular—to concentrate just on carbohydrates or just on protein—cannot compensate for years of bad eating habits. For one thing, the no fat or no anything diet is just another kind of excess. It contradicts nature. Take a look at the variety of fresh produce offered at your market even in winter. Given the variety of this earth, can it possibly be natural, or healthful, or good for you, to eat only pineapple or low-fat cottage cheese for weeks at a time?

Third, as for nutrition in a capsule, it is not only ineffective, it may be dangerous. In the 1980s, beta carotene pills were all the rage, promoted vigorously as being effective in preventing cancer and heart disease. A dozen years after beta carotene supplements first appeared in the marketplace, studies demonstrated that they were useless; as one report put it, the supplements had proved "completely ineffective" in preventing disease and were possibly even harmful in some individuals. Instead of supplements, said the experts, get your beta carotene in food—in the fruits and vegetables in which they naturally occur.

The answer, therefore, is no more in the short-run, quick-fix, single-focus deprivation diet than in the search for a magic potion or pill. There is simply no alternative to a fundamental change in long-term diet. It is essential for good health.

The good news is that it is not difficult to make the change to a healthful diet. For at the center of this new way of eating are the PowerFoods, ten groups of fruits, vegetables, grains, legumes, nuts, and seeds in varied color, taste, and texture that can be combined in endless ways to find a place at every meal. The evidence is mounting that the PowerFoods contain substances that just may be, if anything can be, elixirs of long life and good health.

PowerFoods and Phytochemicals

The key substances are phytochemicals—"phyto" is derived from the ancient Greek word for "plant"—which are simply the compounds within plants with a capacity for reaction and interaction. Of course, the nutritional value of plant foods has long been known; scientific studies as well as common-sense observation confirm that people whose diets are rich in fruits and vegetables live healthier lives. Starting back in the 1970s, however, scientists began to explore the specific medicinal benefits of such diets. These studies went beyond the vitamin and mineral content of fruits and vegetables to their phytochemicals—and to how those phytochemicals react with one another.

What scientists found—and are still finding—was that a single fruit or vegetable contains thousands of phytochemicals in trace amounts that interact in complex but complementary ways to prevent certain diseases and boost overall health. It is awesome to think that every bite of apricot, every leaf of a green leafy vegetable, every mushroom contains a rich chemical stew that can, among other things, block, retard, suppress, or flush away carcinogens; lower serum cholesterol and decrease arterial plaque; enhance the immune system; fight the effects of aging.

There are hundreds of different phytochemicals, although only a small percentage have thus far been identified in nutritional laboratories. In fact, these chemical compounds are so new that nutritionists still haven't agreed on a name; I call them phytochemicals, but you may see them called, variously, nutraceuticals, phytomins, phytonutrients, bioactive components, functional foods, even designer foods. Whatever name wins, it may someday be as common as "vitamins" and "minerals."

Even as the research on phytochemicals goes forward, the basic evidence is too easy to miss. So are the benefits of eating the fruits and vegetables in which phytochemicals occur, fruits and vegetables typically available year-round, easy to buy, store, and prepare, delicious to eat. PowerFoods are particularly rich in phytochemicals, and they are particularly powerful against the diseases and conditions that plague us today. They offer benefits *beyond* basic nutrition—what we might call "supranutrition." They do more than provide energy and the building blocks for tissue growth and repair; they actually work proactively to help prevent disease and fight the effects of aging. To understand this "supranutrition," it's important to know what basic nutrition is all about.

The Basic Nutrients

Nutrients are substances that are essential for life. The six basic nutrients are carbohydrates, protein, fat, vitamins, minerals, and water. Humans take in these nutrients through food, and if we are deprived of too many nutrients for too long, we weaken, we become ill, and eventually we die.

Water is the basic nutrient, essential for life, whether the life is human, animal, or plant. More than two-thirds of the human body consists of water—and more than two-thirds of the earth's surface is covered by water.

Of the other five basic nutrients, the carbohydrates, protein, and fat are macronutrients, while vitamins and minerals are micronutrients. The former are called macronutrients because they are essential in large amounts; micronutrients are essential in minute amounts. Both are needed for an organism's proper growth and metabolism. Macronutrients are the "stuff" of the body—its building blocks and energy. Micronutrients trigger the mechanisms that replenish the building blocks and ignite the energy.

Carbohydrates, often colloquially called "carbs," are the body's primary source of energy. They fuel the body—its muscle, brain, and central nervous system. The energy in food is measured in calories, and carbohydrates provide four calories per gram. Excess carbohydrate calories are stored in the liver and muscles as glycogen, to be called up when needed as a reserve energy source, or, if not needed, to become fat deposits.

Protein is essential for creating and repairing vital cells and organs. Protein is created in the body from building blocks known as amino acids. There are twenty-two different amino acids that can be assembled in thousands of combinations to provide just the right proteins for an individual's unique needs for organs, muscle, blood, hormones, and enzymes. Fourteen of these amino acids can be manufactured in the body, but eight so-called "essential" amino acids must be obtained from food. Protein also provides energy, in the amount of four calories per gram.

Fat is a critical component of cell membranes and hormones and is essential to the process by which some nutrients are absorbed into the system. Fat also cushions organs and helps regulate the body temperature by insulating the body. Fat, too, yields energy: nine calories per gram, more than twice the caloric content of carbs and protein. PowerFoods are an excellent source of essential fatty acids, the building blocks of healthy fat.

All the macronutrients—proteins, carbohydrates, and fats—are substances that undergo chemical transformation to sustain and fuel our bodies. The sparkplugs of the transformation—and thus of nutrition—are the micronutrients, the vitamins and minerals. They are essential components of enzymes that light the fuses under the macronutrients, changing the food we eat into heat and energy, and aiding the body in defending itself against harmful substances.

Vitamins do much more than prevent disease. They provide the only source of certain co-enzymes necessary for metabolism, the biochemical processes that support life. In addition, certain vitamins act as *antioxidants*—substances that protect the body's cells from the kind of damage that can be caused by pollution, exposure to chemicals, alcohol, and the by-products of normal metabolism. Antioxidants raid the *free radicals,* the destructive biological molecules that attack cell membranes and cause premature cell death. In their antioxidant role, vitamins are essential in preventing early aging and many of the degenerative diseases.

Minerals are multifunctional within the body, essential to both structure and function. Calcium and phosphorus are components of bones and teeth. Magnesium is needed for cellular metabolism, sodium for fluid balance and muscle function, potassium for fluid-electrolyte and acid–base balance, chloride for water balance and digestion, and sulfur for protein structure and enzyme activity.

It took science some time to develop this understanding of basic nutrition. Diseases like scurvy and beriberi raged for centuries before scientists even theorized that they resulted from nutritional deficiencies. It took decades more before they identified and isolated the vitamins and minerals that were deficient. In fact, it wasn't until 1948 that all thirteen vitamins considered essential to human health were isolated.

Phytochemicals, which only came under the microscope in the late twentieth century, play a very different role in nutrition. In fact, phytochemicals are non-nutritives. As the name makes clear, they offer no nutrition *per se,* but they are spark plugs for various actions and behaviors within the body's nutritional system.

In plants, phytochemicals occur in minute amounts—trace amounts, as scientists say—but they interact in complex but complementary ways to fight the stress inflicted on plants by intense sunlight, or by insects, or by fungus or mold, or by virus invasions, or by atmospheric pollution. They actually toughen the cells of the plant to ward off deterioration and toxic influences. It's no coincidence that 25 percent of all prescription drugs are derived from natural plant substances, or that many more drugs are synthetic versions of natural plant chemicals.

Humans encounter invasive viruses just as plants do, and we, too, can be made very sick and weak by stress and pollution. The illnesses that result from these problems take a variety of forms: hypertension, cardiovascular sickness, arthritis, gastrointestinal disorders, cancer, and more. Phytochemicals in the plant foods we eat can provide the same health benefits to humans that they provide to plants. Beyond the body-building, body-sustaining power of macronutrients, beyond the sparkplug capabilities of the micronutrients, phytochemicals provide essential raw materials for suppressing, retarding, even reversing not just illnesses but also the debilitating effects of stressful contemporary life and the degenerative effects of aging.

PowerFoods

Putting PowerFoods First

It would be foolish to ignore the evidence emerging from prestigious scientific laboratories all over the world. And it would be silly indeed to spurn the "elixir of life"—if anything deserves the name—so close at hand, the PowerFoods.

This book is about putting PowerFoods first in a rich and varied diet that can sustain and satisfy every hunger and every taste. I have sorted the PowerFoods into ten categories that have now been associated with the prevention and treatment of at least four of the leading causes of death in this country—cardiovascular disease, cancer, hypertension, and diabetes—as well as with the prevention and treatment of such ailments as arthritis, osteoporosis, gastrointestinal disorders, even some of the harsher symptoms of menopause.

In addition to these potential healing benefits, a diet that puts these "top ten" PowerFoods first can make you feel and look better. Studies have shown that a diet dominated by PowerFoods boosts all-around well-being. On a PowerFoods-based diet, people have lost weight, felt better, and reported improved skin tone, thicker hair, stronger nails, and increased vitality and energy.

Since the beneficial effects of phytochemicals are best realized naturally rather than synthetically, putting PowerFoods first is about real food, not pills. There is no evidence that phytochemicals as supplements have anything like the power of whole foods. Rather, what plant biologists are discovering is that any one vegetable or fruit may have thousands of biologically active phytochemicals. Every bite of a PowerFood is a cocktail containing thousands of these phytochemicals, all of them acting together in mysterious ways to offer a multitude of effects, fighting against the likes of cancer and heart disease while bestowing good health and vitality.

From sweet treat fruits like figs to pungent, robust workhorses like garlic, in all their diverse textures, odors, tastes, and in a rainbow of color, the power of these plant foods is in the way the phytochemicals combine. When they do so, they ignite a synergy of pharmacological activity where the whole is greater than the sum of the parts. It is only by eating the whole foods that you can benefit from the process at work inside your body.

As a physician, I know that a way of eating that focuses on PowerFoods is far more in tune with our biology than the typical American diet today. The fact is that humans are genetically programmed to digest and assimilate PowerFoods; that is what our natural metabolism was built for. PowerFoods put less stress on the body, requiring less effort for digestion and assimilation even as they put more energy, more good health into the body.

There is no guarantee against disease, of course. Genetics, behavior, and the luck of the draw all play a part. But the verdict is in: What we eat determines to a great extent how we feel and how well we fight illness and physical decline. When PowerFoods dominate our diet, we give ourselves the best chance for health, well-being, and a vigorous longevity. It really is time—past time, as the second millennium approaches—for Americans to change the way they eat.

The PowerFoods

These are the top ten groups of food that will create and sustain health. Combinations of these—which appear in the recipes—are easy to prepare and delicious to eat:

o **Red, yellow, and orange fruits**
o **Red, yellow, and orange vegetables**
o **Cruciferous and leafy green vegetables**
o **Mushrooms**
o **Sea vegetables**
o **Garlic and company**
o **Whole grains**
o **Beans and other legumes**
o **Soy and soy products**
o **Nuts and seeds**

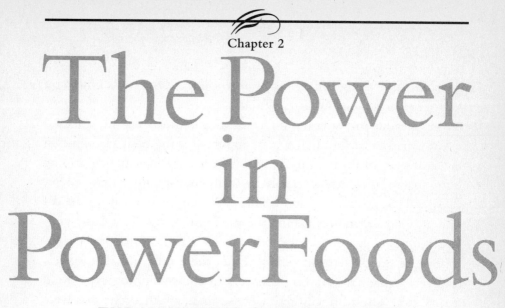

Chapter 2

The Power in PowerFoods

THE MOUNTING EVIDENCE ABOUT PHYTOCHEMICALS

Eat five different kinds of fruits and vegetables every day to recapture the disease-preventing phytochemicals missing in the American diet. Taking vitamin and mineral pills will not prevent the diseases associated with a processed-food diet. Scientists cannot formulate into pills nutrients they haven't yet discovered.
—DR. JAMES DUKE, U.S. DEPARTMENT OF AGRICULTURE

Never before has the focus on the health benefits of commonly available foods been so strong. The philosophy that food can be health-promoting beyond its nutritional value is gaining acceptance within the public arena and among the scientific community as mounting research links diet/food components to disease prevention and treatment.
—POSITION OF THE AMERICAN DIETETIC ASSOCIATION ON PHYTOCHEMICALS

*i*ndoles. Sulforaphanes. Carotenoids. Protease inhibitors. Coumarins. Fatty acids. Flavonoids. Monoterpenes. Isothiocyanates.

These tongue-twisting phytochemicals are the most exciting

things to come along in the nutrition world in a long time. Nutrition as a science originated in the twentieth century. It is a work in progress, one that steadily increases our understanding of how we assimilate food and how particular foods affect just about all of the body's systems. In the early years of the century, scientists deepened their understanding of the macronutrients, primarily by studying how their deficiencies weakened the immune system. The 1920s and thirties were breakthrough years for understanding the micronutrients, as the basic vitamins and minerals were discovered, identified, and isolated.

One of the bizarre side effects of all these nutritional advances, however, was corresponding progress in the technologies of food preservation. The advances here were so dramatic that scientists were able to go beyond preserving foods to actually create new foods altogether—wholly artificial or "junk" foods, touted as another important time-saver for a democracy on the move. Eventually, it was jokingly said, science would be capable of creating foods that had absolutely no nutritional value whatsoever. It was no joke. Obesity became one of the new diseases of the age—malnutrition manifested not in skinniness but in extreme overweight.

Coupled with this bleak nutritional picture were the stresses and strains of life in the twentieth century and the impact of such conditions as overcrowding and pollution. The result was the grim health statistics—*ill* health statistics—cited at the beginning of this book.

In the last years of the twentieth century, a steady barrage of nutritional discoveries has revealed why certain foods help and others hinder the body's functioning and its ability to ward off disease. The late 1980s and 1990s were the breakthrough years for phytochemicals. In 1989, a study investigating occurrence of second primary cancers came up with an interesting finding: that the risk of second primary cancers was 40 to 60 percent lower among patients whose diet had emphasized dark green leafy vegetables, legumes, cruciferous and yellow vegetables, and fresh fruits. Of course, people had always known these foods were "good for you," but that these particular foods should be associated with these particular cancer-fighting statistics raised a flag.

Nutritional scientists set out to discover why such a diet seemed to prevent disease. Thus began the ongoing search for and identification of phytochemical after phytochemical after phytochemical. Throughout the nineties, research results poured in from all over the world: At Cornell University, researchers isolated the sulforaphanes in cruciferous vegetables, showing them to be effective in preventing cancer. In Cairo, the essential fatty acids in pumpkin-seed oil were shown to be effective against arthritic inflammation. At Harvard Medical School, it was shown that the lycopenes in tomatoes lowered the risk of prostate cancer. In Hannover, Germany, a study on flavonoids showed that they helped prevent gastrointestinal diseases. In Rome, quercetins were shown to inhibit the growth of acute leukemias. In Ontario, Canada, the alpha-linolenic acid and lignans in flax seed were shown to be a potential treatment for lupus nephritis.

More and more studies brought more and more good news about phytochemicals from the front lines of the battle against disease. Foremost among the pioneers in phytochemical research was the National Cancer Institute, which launched a multimillion-dollar project to find, isolate, and study phytochemicals, thus lending even greater support, in money and encouragement, to the search for knowledge about these substances.

What we do know about the power of phytochemicals to fight diseases in humans starts with what we know about the power they exert in the plants in which they naturally occur. Imagine back to the very beginnings of life on earth, when plants lived in a world that had no oxygen at all. As they evolved, they began processing carbon dioxide into energy and releasing oxygen as a by-product. In doing so, however, plants were also polluting their own environment. At the same time, the solar radiation that was necessary for this oxygen-emitting process—the process we call photosynthesis—was itself oxidizing. The sun's exposure could—it still can—cause a loss of electrons, or change an element, or destroy it. Plants *had to* develop defenses against the free radicals of unstable oxygen that threatened their survival. The result was the phytochemicals—vividly hued antioxidants whose presence is announced by a plant's bright color. In protecting the plant from oxidation, the phytochemicals allow photosynthesis to proceed benignly and effectively.

That protective capability of phytochemicals in plants extends also to drought and cold; phytochemicals toughen a plant's cells to withstand such extremes. It extends to toxic pollutants and infestation, against which the phytochemicals serve as enzyme blockers and enhancers. Faced by an invasion of gypsy moths, for example, oak trees produce more tannin as a protection against defoliation. By helping shield a plant from destructive forces, phytochemicals enhance the plant's overall health.

Phytochemicals offer the same protection to the creatures that eat plants—from the rabbit munching on the leaves of wild broccoli to the toddler eating her spinach because her mother tells her she must. Phytochemicals help humans fend off cancer, reduce heart disease, improve strength and energy, and bestow longevity by neutralizing the free radicals. Free radicals are loose cannons—specifically, they are molecules with unstable electrons—that destroy cells by damaging their membranes. When that happens, the cells cease to function properly; they can no longer divide or reproduce. Nutrients can't get in; toxic waste can't get out. The cells steadily decrease in number; the tissues eventually lose their ability to function.

Some of this loss of function is visible. We see it in rougher, less elastic skin—in the wrinkles of aging, the loss of skin tone, the brittle look of hair and nails in the elderly. Some of it is invisible damage—the rigid, calcified arteries that slow us to a painful crawl, the rampaging mutant cells that literally eat away at our bodies. This is the damage that kills us. Often—too often—it kills us slowly and very painfully. Phytochemicals arrest this kind of damage. They wield antioxidants that scavenge the free radicals and prevent them from damaging cells.

Preventing and Fighting Cancer

Cancer is one of the most dreaded of the diseases of this century. Now, at least 200 epidemiological studies from around the world have found a link between a plant-rich diet and a lower risk for many types of cancer. An analysis of data from twenty-three studies found that a diet rich in vegetables and grains slashed colon cancer risk by 40 percent. Another study found that women who ate few vegetables had a 25 percent higher incidence of breast cancer than those who consumed more fresh produce. When the Division of Epidemiology at the University of Minnesota conducted an exhaustive review of the evidence on cancer risk and fruits and vegetables, its researchers found that "from 10 to 70 percent of all cancer is attributable to diet."

The scientists at Minnesota spelled it out:

> *Consumption of carrots and green leafy vegetables is particularly associated with a lower risk of lung cancer. Cruciferous vegetables and carrots are associated with a lower risk of colon cancer. . . . Fruit appears to be strongly associated with lower risk of head and neck cancers. Several vegetables and fruits have been found quite consistently associated with lower risk of stomach cancer, fruit and lettuce in particular. For pancreatic cancer, almost every case-control study has reported that consumption of one or more plant foods is associated with lower risk. . . . Intake of vegetables and fruits in general, and of carrots in particular, is inversely associated with bladder cancer.* *

The reason is the complex interactions and differing but complementary mechanisms of the thousands of phytochemicals present at the same time in plant foods. Each phytochemical acts in its own way to offer a specific disease-protective effect. But when phytochemicals act *together,* their power to keep cell chemistry stable is augmented synergistically, and so is their power to protect and sustain life.

What this means is that at every step along the path toward cancer formation, some phytochemical—or some interaction among phytochemicals, or some mechanism of action resulting from the presence of several phytochemicals—works to retard or block the action of the carcinogens.

Think of a medieval fortress town. To invade it, an enemy must overcome a series of obstacles—an open plain, then a moat, then a palisade of pointed pickets, then another ditch, a thick wall, and so on. Throughout the battle, defenders inside the town must continually devise new tactics of counterattack, one after the other, repulsing each

*Potter, J.D. and Steinmetz, K.A. "There is more to vegetables and fruit than antioxidants and fiber." Division of Epidemiology, University of Minnesota, Proceedings of the Annual Meeting Am. Assoc. Res.; 35:673–4 1994; article number UI9560623.

sortie by the attackers, and sometimes repulsing several attacks at once. Our bodies are the fort, and phytochemicals are our defenders. If carcinogens breach one defense, there are still other ways they can be stopped.

For example, tomatoes, peppers, pineapple, strawberries, and carrots contain tens of thousands of phytochemicals—among them, p-coumaric acid and chlorogenic acid. These two stop the formation of cancer-causing substances by preventing nitric oxide from hooking up with amines, which are components of proteins. Why is that desirable? Because when nitric oxide combines with amines, the result is the formation of nitrosamines, and nitrosamines cause cancer.

Tomatoes and red grapefruit contain lycopene, a prominent promoter of cell differentiation. Cancer cells are undifferentiated; that is, they grow uninhibited by the body's natural controls to become destructive tumors. In northern Italy, where people consume seven or more servings of tomatoes per week, researchers have found as much as a 60 percent lower risk of cancers of the mouth, esophagus, stomach, colon, and rectum. They attribute this astonishing result to lycopene—really, to those luscious plum tomatoes that are almost a staple of northern Italian cuisine.

So tomatoes—and the other red, yellow, and orange PowerFoods—keep carcinogens from forming in the first place; they hold carcinogens at bay.

If carcinogens do form, the phytochemicals we have stocked up on by eating PowerFoods have defensive responses for them. Some phytochemicals work to kick carcinogens out of the cells they have entered. Researchers have determined that sulforaphane keeps living animals from getting cancer by boosting the production of anticancer enzymes—phase-2 eynzmes. These enzymes detoxify carcinogens by hooking them up to molecules that wheel them right out of the cell before they can cause harm. Where does this powerful cancer fighter occur? Sulforaphane is found in broccoli, brussels sprouts, turnips, kale, cauliflower, and other cruciferous vegetables. Simply put, we can say that just by eating tomatoes, we help keep carcinogens from forming; by eating broccoli, we can send them spinning out of the cell.

Still another line of defense is to neutralize carcinogens before

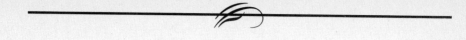

they can invade the cell's DNA and cause mutations. For this, the ellagic acid in strawberries, grapes, and raspberries, and the isothiocyanates in cabbage, turnips, and other crucifers are particularly potent.

If these outside-the-wall defenses should fail, phytochemicals have recourse to other tactics. For example, there is always the possibility of cutting off the supply lines to carcinogens—the tiny capillaries through which oxygen and nutrients reach the mutated cell and nourish the tumor. Genistein, a phytochemical isolated from soybeans, prevents these vital lifelines from forming.

There is dramatic evidence about the consumption of soy foods—not the soy sauce with which Americans typically dress food, but the tofu, tempeh, and whole soybean that are staples of the Japanese diet. When Japanese who move to the West go from their soy-rich diet to an American soy-poor diet, they exhibit much higher rates of breast cancer and prostate cancer than their compatriots who remain at home. The likely reason is the high content of isoflavones, especially genistein, in soy foods. In addition to containing genistein, soy is a complete protein; it contains all the essential amino acids, but unlike animal protein, soy has cholesterol-lowering effects.

Phytochemicals can do more than defend against cancer; they can also counterattack. Indol–3-carbinol, found in cabbage, cauliflower, and other cruciferous vegetables, triggers enzymes that keep the form of estrogen linked to breast cancer from predominating. Allylic sulfide, a phytochemical found in onions and garlic, enhances enzymes that detoxify carcinogens. Capsaicin, in hot chile peppers, and other phytochemicals in such spices as turmeric and cumin, keeps toxic molecules from attaching to DNA and perhaps initiating cancer. Diallyl disulfide blocks and suppresses cancer agents, *and* it stimulates production of a detoxification enzyme called glutathione-S-transferase. You find it in onions, leeks, scallions, chives, shallots, and, most powerfully of all, in garlic. Lignans in flax seeds, barley, and wheat are antioxidants that attack cell-damaging free radicals. Terpenes in citrus fruits increase the production and activation of a protein that interrupts the undifferentiated, out-of-control growth of breast-cancer cells in rats. Phytosterols in whole grains, legumes, and soy quite literally compete with the estrogens that promote cancer; while they don't destroy these cancer-causing agents, they do deflect them from their path. Flavonoids in just about all fruits and vegetables—and in wine—block carcinogens' access to cells and suppress malignant changes in cells.

The obvious conclusion is that the more phytochemicals there are defending us, the stronger our various lines of defense against cancer. The more varied the phytochemicals defending us, the more opportunities there are for the cancer-preventing mechanisms to act. Simply put, PowerFoods are a strong defense against cancer, and a varied stew of PowerFoods is our best ammunition.

HOW THE PHYTOCHEMICALS IN POWERFOODS FIGHT CANCER

Scientists have identified numerous mechanisms of phytochemical action against cancer. Specifically, phytochemicals:

➤ Prevent the formation of carcinogens from precursor substances

➤ Block carcinogens from reaching critical target sites

➤ Suppress cells that have been exposed to carcinogens from turning malignant

➤ Stimulate enzymes that detoxify carcinogens and flush them from the body

➤ Trigger enzymes that block or suppress cellular DNA damage

➤ Inhibit the growth of new blood vessels to nascent tumors from proliferating

➤ Block cellular receptor sites for natural hormones like estrogen that might trigger malignancy

➤ Enhance the immune function

➤ Inhibit enzymes that break down collagen (the glue that holds cells together)

➤ Function as antioxidants to sweep out free radicals

PowerFoods and Heart Health

The term *heart disease* embraces a number of conditions, but the term *heart health* means strong, smooth, elastic, unobstructed arteries capable of responding to numerous variations in blood pressure. Damaged arteries tend to accumulate plaque—that is, deposits of fatty material—at the point of damage; they then lose elasticity, tighten up, and interfere with blood flow. If a clot forms at the site of obstruction and blocks a coronary artery, the result can be a heart attack.

To keep a heart healthy, therefore, it's important to keep the lining of the arteries smooth and undamaged so plaque can't form. And while there are many contributors to the formation of plaque, and many steps to the development of heart disease, we do know that while high-density lipoproteins (HDL) can be beneficial, low-density lipoproteins (LDL), the so-called "bad cholesterol," is dangerous to the heart when it is oxidized by free radicals. In fact, there is considerable evidence that free radicals both directly and indirectly damage arterial walls; the results can be hypertension, atherosclerosis, and strokes.

It makes sense, then, to eat foods rich in antioxidants. The red, green, yellow, and orange PowerFoods are loaded with carotenoids—especially beta-carotene and lycopene—that have been shown to reduce the accumulation of plaque in arteries. One wide-ranging, long-term study confirmed that increased intake of fruit, vegetable, and cereal fiber lowered the risk of coronary heart disease among men by lowering cholesterol and producing "other beneficial physiological effects."[*]

Raw onion, with its high content of organosulfurs—particularly diallyl disulfide—is a potent inhibitor of cholesterol synthesis. Onion, garlic, and all the smelly members of the allium family are PowerFoods important to heart health. The smell comes from the organosulfurs, so it really is an indication of the pharmacological power of these foods to act as antioxidants. For heart health, the power works to reduce buildups in the blood and increase the fluidity of membranes. Studies on garlic in Russia, China, and Japan have shown that it acts much like aspirin to thin the blood and prevent clots. It has also been shown to lower blood pressure.

Anti-Infection Warriors

"We are discovering that some nutriments can be used, not so much as foods, but as modulators, manipulators or stimulators of the immune system," says Dr. Robert A. Good, immunologist and pediatrician at All Childrens Hospital in St. Petersburg, Florida. As anti-infection warriors, PowerFoods can be, in the doctor's words, "pretty powerful medicine."[†]

*Rimm, Eric B. et al., "Vegetable, Fruit, and Cereal Fiber Intake," JAMA, February 14, 1996, Vol 275, No. 6.
†Good, Dr. Robert A., quoted in Encyclopedia Britannica USA Instant Research Service, R–2262.

Increasingly, scientists in the lab and physicians in the sickroom are confirming that manipulating diet can decrease the risk of infection. It has worked for postoperative patients, for burn victims, among the very young and the very old. The research is even showing that diet can be used to retard the aging of the body's immune system, and thus to stave off the diseases and ailments that result from immunological decline.

It's the dark green leafy vegetables, the yellow fruits and vegetables, the allium bulb vegetables, and the whole-grain foods in particular that seem to affect the immune system. The phytochemicals in these foods—allicin, omega–3 fatty acids, and flavonoids—stimulate the white blood cells that bind to invaders, act as antioxidants, and block virus and fungus. They are powerful anti-infection warriors.

Defying Diabetes

A difficult enough disease on its own, diabetes is also a major risk factor for various other diseases—vascular disease, kidney disease, hypertension, blindness. The diabetic is unable to process sugar properly; when the sugar in the bloodstream is elevated high enough, serious problems can result.

Uncontrolled diabetes is extremely serious, and anyone diagnosed with diabetes should be under the care of a physician. But diet is a key therapy for controlling diabetes, as the attending physician will insist, and a diabetic can participate in the management of the disease by eating a variety of PowerFoods.

The phytochemicals, fiber, and low calorie levels of PowerFoods help lower blood sugar and may decrease a diabetic's need for medication. In addition, the same foods that protect so well against heart disease will work to keep diabetes at bay, lowering bad cholesterol and keeping the blood vessels open and smooth. The quercetin in such PowerFoods as citrus, grapes, and most vegetables has proven effective in countering the eye damage that can result from diabetes. Medical anthropologist John Heinerman, in his *Encyclopedia of Fruits, Vegetables, and Herbs,* lists ten foods and two herbs that have been shown to be effective against diabetes—from blueberries, rich in the phytochemical called myrillin, to garlic and onions, so rich in infection-fighting substances called organosulfurs that they are seemingly omnipotent healing foods.* Traditional Chinese medicine also prescribes mushrooms, carrots, wheat bran, corn, and a tea made from dried guava leaves—in addition to garlic and onions—as diabetes fighters.

Answering Arthritis

In the teeth of widespread skepticism, the evidence is mounting that diet has an effect on arthritis. Folk remedies for the painful inflammation of rheumatoid arthritis and the frayed surfaces of the joints in osteoarthritis have long included plants, and science is now telling us that the phytochemicals in peppers—including hot chili peppers, nuts and seeds, and spices are indeed effective against arthritis. One suspected reason is that the heat of the capsaicin in peppers and spices simply shuts down the communication system so that the pain signals cannot get to the brain. In fact, Heinerman reports on research by the U.S. Navy to explore a possible use for capsaicin foods in dealing with so-called "phantom limb pain," the pain that amputees claim to feel in their absent limbs.

In addition to pepper-hot foods, the flavonoids occurring in such fruits and vegetables as citrus, onions, apples, grapes, and tea inhibit certain enzymes that can go out of control and actually destroy such components of the joint as cartilage and bone. They help circulation. And they help return flexibility to joints by restoring collagen.

Gastrointestinal Health

The typical American diet, with its emphasis on meat, dairy, and fat, is especially hard on the gastrointestinal tract. In addition, our possibly excessive intake of antibiotics and anti-inflammatory medications tends to further disrupt the gastrointestinal ecology. When that happens, the normally beneficial bacteria in the gastrointestinal tract are overwhelmed by bad bacteria that damage the integrity of the gas-

*Heinerman, John, *Heinerman's Encyclopedia of Fruits, Vegetables and Herbs.* Parker Publishing Company, Inc., West Nyack, NY. 1988.

trointestinal lining. The lining then leaks toxins and partially digested particles into the bloodstream, where they travel and wreak havoc—everything from asthma to arthritis to chronic fatigue to muscle weakness.

In addition to these far-flung symptoms, the gastrointestinal tract itself can become a target organ for disease; some symptoms are chronic constipation, hemorrhoids, diarrhea, irritable bowel, spastic colon, even colon cancer, one of the most prevalent cancers in "advanced" Western societies.

A PowerFoods diet, with its high fiber content, normalizes elimination of wastes, which helps alleviate these symptoms. Plant foods can ensure normal bacteria. Normal bacteria in turn form a protective barrier in the gastro-intestinal tract and are themselves essential to the body's manufacture of its own beneficial phytochemicals—particularly, the essential fatty acids, or EFAs.

The PowerFoods File: Feeling Fit, Looking Good

When you can prevent, treat, or reverse degenerative diseases, you contribute to your overall fitness and sense of well-being. Beyond this, however, both the lessons of experience and the scientific evidence indicate that putting PowerFoods first makes you feel better and improves your appearance. Eating PowerFoods means maintaining peak energy, a healthy weight, strong brain power, and a calm mental state—as well as disease prevention and anti-aging power. A study I performed with a group of 15-year-old girls at a local high school demonstrated this dramatically.

The girls were all overweight and lived mostly on candy bars, soft drinks, potato chips, and an occasional piece of fried chicken. The experiment put all the girls on a PowerFoods diet and half of them on a regime of monitored exercise three times a week. As expected, there was greater weight loss with the group that exercised, but all the girls realized the benefits of a varied PowerFoods diet. After four weeks on fruits, vegetables, legumes, grains, nuts and seeds—a diet that turned out to be just as convenient as fast food—all the girls lost weight. In addition, their skin cleared up, their hair—an object of great interest to them all—became more lustrous. Their personalities became sunnier and calmer, and they had far fewer visits to the school nurse with minor complaints. Six months later, they were maintaining their PowerFoods diet and were doing well—not because of any concern over preventing cancer or heart disease, but because they felt and looked so good.

Women are learning that putting PowerFoods first can combat the syndrome of varied afflictions known as premenstrual syndrome, PMS. Considerable research has shown that eliminating meat and dairy and significantly increasing PowerFoods in your diet can have a major influence on some of the symptoms of PMS, particularly bloating, breast tenderness, and mood swings. Studies on menopausal women show that the bioflavonoids found in large quantities in green leafy vegetables, in cruciferous vegetables, and in fruits, as well as the isoflavones in soy, act as weak estrogens to relieve or prevent the symptoms of menopause.

The bioflavonoids also have a unique ability to bond to collagen, the glue that holds human cells together, and to inhibit the enzymes that break down collagen. Eating PowerFoods rich in bioflavonoids can help return flexibility to the skin, the arteries, capillaries, joints, and other tissues by restoring collagen. That means they help stave off the wrinkles of age. Moreover, unlike most other known nutrients, the beneficial effects of bioflavonoids cross the blood barrier to the brain where they protect the blood vessels from oxidation, thus showing promise in warding off the ravages of senility.

The power of PowerFoods, in short, is not just their ability to prevent infection, to block cell mutation, to reduce plaque. Their power is also in their ability to enhance vitality and well-being. And that, in turn, can make you look better and feel better about yourself.

Phytochemicals Chart

Phytochemicals	Their Source	Their Power
Carotenoids (over 600) especially beta carotene, lycopene	Red, green, yellow, orange fruits and vegetables especially carrots, sweet potatoes, winter squash, tomatoes, citrus, melons, cruciferous vegetables	Antioxidants; reduce accumulation of plaque in arteries; promote cell differentiation (cancer cells are undifferentiated).
Flavonoids (over 800) especially rutin, hesperidin, and quercetin	Most fruits and vegetables, especially citrus, onions, apples, grapes, tea	Antioxidants that block carcinogens, suppress malignant changes, keep collagen healthy. Protect eyes, nerves from inflammation and damage from diabetes: improve symptoms of allergy, asthma, and arthritis.
Ellagic acid	Strawberries, grapes, raspberries, apples	Neutralize cancer-causing chemicals found in tobacco smoke, processed foods, and barbecued meats.
Phenolic acids	Citrus, whole grains, berries, tomatoes, peppers, parsley, carrots, cruciferous vegetables, squash, yams, most other fruits and vegetables	Help resist cancer by inhibiting cell proliferation induced by carcinogens in target organs; inhibit platelet activity, decrease inflammation, and act as antioxidants.
Indoles	Cruciferous vegetables, such as broccoli, cabbage, kale	Block cancer-causing substances before they can damage cells.

Phytochemicals	Their Source	Their Power
Isothiocyanates, such as sulforaphane	Cruciferous vegetables	Induce protective enzymes; suppress tumor growth.
Lignans	Flax seeds, berries, whole grains	Antioxidants and insoluble fibers; block or suppress cancerous changes; anti-inflammatory; particularly protective against colon cancer and heart disease.
Saponins	Garlic, onions, legumes, soybeans	Inhibit tumor promoters induced by excessively fatty diet; lower circulating levels of fats.
Protease inhibitors	All plants, especially soybeans	Reduce inflammation of arthritis; antiviral and antibacterial; suppress enzyme production in cancer cells, which may slow tumor growth.
Terpenes	Oranges, lemons, grapefruit	Induce protective enzymes; interfere with the action of carcinogens; prevent dental decay; antiulcer activity.
Capsaicin	Hot peppers	Reduce pain sensation; anti-inflammatory; prevents the activation of cancer-causing chemicals.

Phytochemicals	Their Source	Their Power
Coumarins	Soybeans, whole grains, citrus, cruciferous vegetables, cucumbers, squash, melons, parsley, flax seeds, green tea	Anticancer activists; blood thinners.
Isoflavones, such as genistein, daidzein	Soybeans, tofu, soy milk	Antioxidants that block carcinogens, suppress tumor formation; block estrogen from entering cells to reduce risk of breast and ovarian cancer.
Organosulfurs, such as allicin, diallyl disulfide	Garlic, onions, leeks, chives, shallots, scallions	Block or suppress cancer-causing agents; inhibit cholesterol synthesis; boost immunity; prevent infection. Help resist cancer by inhibiting nitrosamine formation and interfering with cancer-causing enzymes.
Phytosterols	Whole grains, legumes, soy	Compete with natural estrogens that may promote cancer.

Chapter 3

Putting PowerFoods First

A WAY OF EATING FOR
THE TWENTY-FIRST CENTURY

The dietary evidence continues to support our recommendations to eat a diet rich in vegetables, fruits, and whole grains. There appears to be practically no limit to the health benefits of such a diet.
—GEOFFREY CANNON, PH.D. SCIENCE DIRECTOR
WORLD CANCER RESEARCH FUND

Vitamin and mineral supplements are no substitute for a variety of foods. Because fruits, vegetables, and grains contain a synergistic mix of micronutrients that hasn't been duplicated in pills or capsules, eating a wide range of foods from the plant kingdom is considered better than relying on supplements.
—DIETARY GUIDELINES FOR AMERICANS
U.S. DEPARTMENT OF AGRICULTURE

given what we know about the relationship between diet and health, given the growing body of long-term studies and the mounting discoveries from laboratories, given what scientific authorities and our own common sense tell us, isn't it time for a change in the way we eat?

The world is full of a wondrous variety of pleasures (among them, eating) and of a wondrous variety of foods. It would be foolish, and contrary to nature, to deprive yourself of all this wonder, or to abandon some tastes or textures, or to relinquish favorite dishes. There is no need to do so; in fact, it's a bad idea. The widened horizon is not just pleasing to the palate; it is absolutely essential to the body's health. Some of the PowerFoods in this book may be new to you—specifically, sea vegetables. Try them. It's never too late to develop new tastes, especially with so much at stake.

Be more adventurous with the old tastes, too. If you eat broccoli regularly, try such other dark green leafies as kale, collards, and beet greens. Or, add sweet potatoes, tomatoes, red peppers, mushrooms, or nuts to your favorite broccoli recipe. Become an artist of PowerFoods and widen the palette of colors you feed your palate. Mix it up. To the basic greens, add some of the wonderful reds: beets and peppers, strawberries and cherries. Brighten a red and green combination with oranges and yellows: carrots and sweet potatoes, lemons and squashes. Experiment. The ways you find to put PowerFoods first are limited only by your creativity and imagination. Remember the seasons. Use herbs and spices liberally in your menu planning and meal preparation. All herbs and spices are beneficial foods and are important to a PowerFoods diet. Spices tend to be extremely rich in phytochemicals, and the healing powers of herbs are well-known. That's why herbs and spices are highlighted in our recipes even though present in small amounts.

Eat less, but perhaps more frequently. Humans started off as gatherers, grazing among the plants of the earth, nibbling a little from this fruit, a little from that vegetable. Perhaps it's time to return to that kind of sampling variety. While we would never wish to return to an era of depending for survival on what we can find, we would do well to copy that formula of eating small quantities of a great variety of foods.

Enjoy all things in moderation. Calorie-counting, gram-measuring, and ingredient analysis are *immoderate,* detracting from the pleasure of food. Different people achieve their nutritional needs in different ways, sometimes planning ahead, sometimes compensating later. The overriding principle is to eat PowerFoods in greater proportions than you eat anything else.

The key that opens the door to variety *and* moderation is balance. In 1990, the same year a new set of dietary guidelines for health was issued by the government, a select group of noted health professionals and culinary experts got together to explore ways to convince people that good food and good health are not mutually exclusive. The meeting, called Resetting the American Table, represented a unique look at nutrition as a matter of taste. The result was that the attendees embraced the new dietary guidelines and added two of their own: First, *all* foods can be part of a healthful diet when considered over time; and second, with a little planning, a diet can include foods of high- as well as moderate- or low-fat content and still meet dietary guidelines.

That's why the recipes in this book include such ingredients as dairy products and meat, both high in animal protein and fat. After all, Parmesan cheese is what gives that special kick to the Pasta with Zucchini Sauce (page 282); lamb provides the robust flavor of the Root Vegetables and Lamb Stew (page 283); chicken stock enhances many of the soup recipes. In adopting the PowerFoods principle, the idea is not to say farewell forever to non-PowerFoods. In fact, the non-PowerFoods can give special taste or texture to a dish, and taste and texture are important.

The heart of the matter is to evaluate diet over a period of time—several days, even weeks—rather than by individual foods or meals. Evaluating over time lets you plan ahead for or make up after special occasions, and that in turn lets you enjoy your favorites foods—a special dessert, for example, or a big meal—without the guilt that is often associated with such indulgence. And guilt, like certain foods, is bad for your health.

What's *good* for your health is to enjoy all the abundant generosity of nature, including favorite foods. Forget the balanced meal and start planning the balanced diet, a way of eating that puts life-style in balance with the human metabolism and benefits both in the process. Not surprisingly, after you have done so for a while, you will begin to *crave* PowerFoods first; the PowerFoods discipline becomes the natural thing to do, as indeed it is.

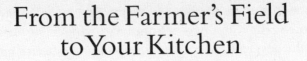

From the Farmer's Field
to Your Kitchen

In the beginning, fruits and vegetables grew wild. Over time, our forebears found that parts of these plants were edible—leaves, flowers, buds, stalks, roots, bulbs, fruits, seeds—and eventually, humans learned to cultivate these plants for use as human and animal food. Cultivation didn't become a science, however, until the agricultural revolution of the sixteenth and seventeenth centuries, while plant breeding and the science of agronomy are even more recent developments.

These developments, coupled with progress in transportation, refrigeration, and food preservation, have had the happy result of enabling Americans to obtain an ever-expanding variety of fresh PowerFoods just about any time of the year. Many of these fruits and vegetables are a far cry from their wild forebears; they have been produced by genetic engineering techniques perfected over the centuries. They widen the pool and extend the availability of PowerFoods.

The trade-off for this volume and variety, however, and for the year-round availability, is that modern, large-scale farming tends to emphasize crops with a stalwart, robust constitution. That means breeding for toughness, the use of chemicals to kill crop-damaging insects, and various methods of handling to ensure that the fruits and vegetables will survive a trip from California's Imperial Valley to a supermarket in your town or city. Taste and texture are often lost.

Moreover, the use of pesticides (and the freshness-maintaining waxes that often lock in pesticides) is a matter of concern to many people. In this regard, it is worth remembering that plants themselves create "pesticide" protection all the time; antioxidants, after all, are a defense system against unstable forms of oxygen, while the ethylene gas that ripe fruits naturally emit is actually an anesthetic.

There is no convincing evidence as yet that the pesticide content of America's vegetable crop is harmful. By the same token, the hardiness that results from large-scale farming methods has no bearing on the nutritional and supranutritional value of these PowerFoods. The best protection in the face of concerns about both taste and toxins is to buy fresh PowerFoods in season and, if possible, locally, and be sure to rinse them carefully in fresh, clear water. You are better off eating PowerFoods that may have been treated with pesticides than not eating PowerFoods at all.

The PowerFood Kitchen: Tools of the Trade

Putting PowerFoods first does not require going out and buying fancy equipment or special gadgets. For one thing, for greatest effectiveness, most PowerFoods are best eaten raw—fresh and uncooked. That is certainly true of the fruits and salad greens.

In the PowerFoods kitchen, therefore, the tools of the trade are basic. You probably have most of them already. The following list includes most of the essentials:

- **Vegetable brush**
- **Three sharp knives: a paring knife, a chef's knife, a knife with a serrated edge**
- **Vegetable peeler**
- **Colander**
- **Collapsible metal steamer**
- **Blender**
- **Cutting board**
- **Rubber or plastic spatulas in a range of sizes**
- **Wooden spoons**
- **Lots of storage bags and covered containers**

The fact is, the skins, cores, and interior membranes of fruits and vegetables are nutrient-rich, stockpiled with phytochemicals. The stringy white inner covering between the skin of the orange and its meat; the core of the apple; the pits or seeds of the watermelon, pumpkin, or squash; the casing on the potato: These are treasure-houses of good health and disease prevention.

So whenever possible, when aesthetics and taste factors permit, keep pith and pit out of the compost heap (or garbage disposal). I find that these little scraps make great nibbles during meal preparation.

By the same token, when PowerFoods are cooked, it is better to steam than to boil them; some phytochemicals may be partially destroyed by the heat required in boiling. To steam food in the microwave, use a microwave-safe container. Sprinkle a tablespoon or two of water over the raw PowerFoods in the container. Then cover. Zapping time varies, depending on the vegetable, but count on anywhere from two minutes for peas to as many as fifteen minutes for an artichoke.

Since it is equally possible to steam vegetables in a small metal steamer set in a saucepan of boiling water, a microwave oven might be considered a useful but nonessential tool of the PowerFoods kitchen. Other useful tools are a mini food processor and a maxi food processor.

A mini food processor is useful for chopping—especially for chopping such things as onions and garlic that will then be put in the blender. However, onions and garlic that are headed for the sauté pan will look better and be easier to handle if they are chopped the old-fashioned way with a chef's knife. A maxi processor, on the other hand, will do the work of the mini processor and the blender combined: all the chopping and slicing, all the blending and puréeing you need for everything from salads to pasta sauce to soups.

Incidentally, fresh juices that include pulp from PowerFoods are a nutritional powerhouse. If you have the proper juice extractor, the kind that processes the whole fruit, this is definitely a desirable tool of the trade.

The PowerFoods Pantry

Having a well-stocked pantry and a refrigerator for the perishables lets you whip up a meal or snack quickly and conveniently, even if you have to make a last-minute stop for fresh produce. The list that follows includes ingredients used in our chefs' recipes, as well as some staples of any kitchen. Specific examples—suggestions only—

are in parentheses. Use this list and your imagination to create your own dishes, putting PowerFoods first.

Produce

- ○ **Fresh seasonal fruits and vegetables**
- ○ **Dried fruits and vegetables (apricots, figs, sun-dried tomatoes, mushrooms)**
- ○ **Frozen vegetables (unseasoned, no sauces)**
- ○ **Juice-packed canned fruits**
- ○ **Solid-packed pumpkins, yams, squashes**
- ○ **Canned tomatoes, tomato sauce, tomato paste**
- ○ **Frozen fruits (unsweetened)**
- ○ **100 percent fruit and vegetable juices (fresh or from concentrate)**

Grains

- ○ **Whole grain breads**
- ○ **Pita bread**
- ○ **Low-fat crackers (Finn Crisp, Ry-Krisp, Ak-mak)**
- ○ **Breadsticks**
- ○ **Tortillas (soft—corn, whole wheat, multigrain)**
- ○ **Hot cereals (oats, barley, farina, mixed grains, cream of wheat, cream of rye)**
- ○ **Cold cereals made from whole grains with fewer than eight grams of added sugar per serving**
- ○ **Brown rice, basmati rice**
- ○ **Variety grains (quinoa, millet, barley, kasha, bulgur)**
- ○ **Couscous/pasta in a variety of shapes and flavors**

Legumes

- ○ **Dried peas and lentils**
- ○ **Dried or canned beans**
- ○ **Soy foods: tempeh, tofu (shelf-stable, reduced-fat, and ready-ground tofu are available)**

Nonvegetable Proteins

- ○ Fresh fish fillets
- ○ Fresh or frozen shrimp, crab, lobster
- ○ Fresh scallops, mussels, clams
- ○ Canned water-packed tuna, salmon, sardines
- ○ Skinless, boneless chicken breast or turkey breast
- ○ Ground chicken or turkey breast

Dairy and Non-Dairy

- ○ Skim or 1% milk, skim buttermilk, skim or 1% soy or rice milk
- ○ Nonfat yogurt, plain or with fruit
- ○ Nonfat sour cream
- ○ Fromage blanc
- ○ Evaporated skim milk
- ○ Part-skim or low-fat cheese, soy or almond cheese (5 or fewer grams of fat per ounce of cheese)
- ○ Grated Parmesan, Romano, or soy Parmesan cheese
- ○ Powdered skim milk, dry soy milk powder
- ○ Part-skim or low-fat ricotta, cottage cheese, or cream cheese

Basics, Condiments, Sauces, and Stocks

- ○ Whole wheat flour, unbleached all-purpose flour
- ○ Wheat bran, wheat germ
- ○ Cornmeal
- ○ Sweeteners: molasses, granulated sugar, light/dark brown sugar, honey
- ○ Cornstarch
- ○ Baking soda, baking powder
- ○ Gelatin, unflavored
- ○ Cocoa powder

- Pancake syrup, maple or fruit types
- Fruit "butters" (all-fruit)
- Natural fruit jam (any flavor)
- Jelly for cooking: mint, currant, jalapeño pepper, and others
- Marmalade: orange, ginger, lime, lemon
- Chutney (any flavor)
- Cranberry sauce and/or unsweetened apple sauce
- Mustards: yellow, spicy, honey, Dijon, or others
- Ketchup, chili sauce, cocktail sauce
- Salsa or picante sauce
- Sauces for cooking: barbecue, Tabasco, hoisin, low-sodium soy sauce, tamari
- Horseradish, wasabi powder
- Powdered kelp, sea vegetable flakes
- Green chiles, jalapeños, pimientos
- Pickle relish: pickles, roasted peppers (hot or sweet)
- Vinegars: balsamic, raspberry, white, sherry, cider, rice, wine
- Olives and capers
- Fat-free or low-fat salad dressings/mayonnaise
- Reduced sodium stocks: vegetable, chicken, beef

Nuts, Seeds, and Oils

- Nuts: almonds, walnuts, pecans, chestnuts, pine nuts, hazelnuts, peanuts
- Seeds: caraway, dill, fennel, sesame, poppy, flax, sunflower, pumpkin
- Oils: olive, canola, flax seed, sesame, walnut, peanut
- Nut butters: peanut, almond, sesame (tahini), and the like (look for all-natural or unhomogenized brands)

Herbs, Spices, and Flavorings

- Herbs (fresh or dried): basil, bay leaf, marjoram, oregano, parsley, rosemary, sage, tarragon, thyme, others of choice

- ○ Spices: cinnamon, nutmeg, allspice, cloves, cumin, paprika, pepper, others of choice
- ○ Seasoning powders: chili, curry, garlic, onion, others of choice
- ○ Seasoning blends: Greek, Italian, Mexican, Cajun, Southwestern, others of choice
- ○ Pure extracts: almond, vanilla, orange, mint, others of choice

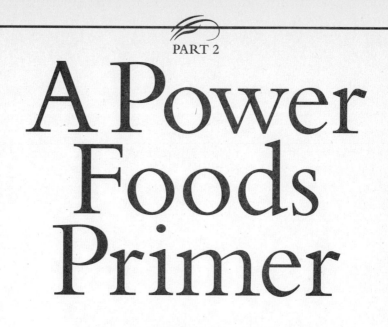

PART 2

A Power Foods Primer

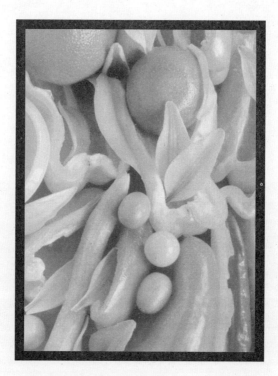

Chapter 4

Red, Yellow, and Orange Fruits

It is unfortunate that Americans are digging their graves with their knives and forks. The refined carbohydrate and processed food diet that many people live on leads to the development of degenerative illnesses as we age—namely, diabetes, arthritis, heart disease, and cancer. Essential to the health of our digestive tract and immune system is to eat a large variety of colorful foods, especially fruits.

—DR. JOEL FUHRMAN,
ST. BARNABAS HOSPITAL, LIVINGSTON, NJ
AUTHOR, *FASTING AND EATING FOR HEALTH*

*P*hytochemicals are brought to you in glorious technicolor. Their brilliant hues paint the plants in which they occur, thus dramatizing their power as fighters against disease and aging. The deeper the color of the plant, the greater the concentration of phytochemicals.

This is vividly evident in the red, yellow, and orange fruits. It is hardly surprising that these PowerFoods have long been inspiration for artists. From the wall paintings in the dining rooms of ancient Roman villas that reproduced the plums, berries, and melons the diners were eating to the cascades of grapes and clusters of bananas represented in the lush canvases of the Renaissance to the bowls of apples and pears depicted in the still lifes of the Impressionists, the fruits of earth, vine, and tree have been regarded as objects of beauty.

All fruits are the matured ovaries—including the seeds—of seed-bearing plants. They are the fulfillment of a long, often laborious process of growth. After this maturity, decay sets in, and the seed within the fruit, perhaps transported by bird, bee, or wind, has a chance to sprout into new life somewhere else.

There are many ways to classify fruits. Botanists speak of four types: simple, aggregate, multiple, and accessory. Simple fruits are the fleshy berries or the so-called drupes like peaches, apricots, nectarines, and plums. Aggregate fruits are a collection of small drupes, each of which has developed from a separate ovary of the same flower—raspberries, for example. Multiple fruits develop from a cluster of ovaries; the pineapple is the classic multiple fruit, a combination of many fruitlets that have bloomed to unite with a single stalk. Accessory fruits are those containing tissue from parts of the plant other than just the ovary; the apple, for example, is actually a swollen stem.

We might classify fruits by the way they grow: on stalks like pineapples and bananas, on vines like grapes and melons, on bushes or brambles like some of the berries, and on trees like everything from apples to cherries to peaches to citrus fruits.

We might even classify fruits by the environment in which they grow and the images they evoke. There are the tropical fruits, like papayas and pineapples, redolent of lush, humid islands brushed by warm ocean breezes. Chilled, these fruits help to cool us when it's hot. Then there are the cool-weather fruits—apples and pears—that hint of crisp coolness; we even think of their color as "autumnal." These fruits lend themselves well to cooking, which is especially nice for fall and winter eating; they fill pies and tarts, and can be baked, glazed, poached, or flambéed.

We can classify fruits by what they wear, by their texture, by how they taste. Some of the red, yellow, and orange fruits have rinds that must be removed before the fruit can be eaten—most notably the orange itself, or how about the watermelon?—while fruits like apples are typically eaten with the skin on.

Melons and papayas are soft-fleshed fruits. The citrus fruits tend to have stringy meat. Pears offer a chewy interior under their thin, tight skins. Grapes pop al dente the way pasta is supposed to.

The tastes of fruits are as varied as these textures, shapes, ways of growing, shades of color. Overall, however, fruits have a sweet taste. Sometimes it is pungent, as in a Granny Smith apple, and sometimes it's mild and sugary, as in a watermelon. Whatever the variation, the theme is a sweet one, giving the lie to the notion that things that taste good can't possibly be good for you. After all, a fruit was the first temptation.

Classifying fruits by color emphasizes their phytochemical content. The rich red fruits—watermelon, raspberries, strawberries, and ruby red grapefruit, for example—are rich in lycopene, a strong antioxidant that scavenges harmful free radicals. The yellow fruits—bananas, lemons, yellow grapefruit, pineapple—often represent a range of phytochemicals, but prominent among the phytochemicals they contain are the antioxidant flavonoids and the cancer-preventing terpenes. The orange fruits—both the ordinary orange and more offbeat specimens like papaya and apricot—are particularly rich in carotenoids, the best known of which is beta carotene.

The Beta Carotene Controversy

Yellow as well as orange fruits contain large stores of beta carotene. Beta carotene is a precursor of Vitamin A; that is, the livers of most mammals manufacture Vitamin A from the beta carotene found in plants. Beta carotene is also one of the trendiest antioxidant discoveries of the 1980s. So exciting were the original findings about it that two studies were undertaken, both financed by the National Cancer Institute, to test whether a beta carotene supplement, in a capsule, might fend off cancer and other diseases.

One study, the Physicians' Health Study, followed 22,071 doctors who were randomly assigned to take a pill of beta carotene or a dummy capsule every other day. The monitoring went on for 12 years. A second study, the Beta Carotene and Retinol Efficacy Trial, tested 18,314 participants, feeding them supplements of beta carotene, Vitamin A, both, or a placebo, also over a period of years. In January, 1996, the results of those studies put a damper on the beta carotene fad. They showed that taking a beta carotene supplement was "completely ineffective," as the announcement phrased it, in preventing cancer or heart disease. What's more, the second study showed that the supplements might actually be harmful. In that study, the incidence of both cancer and heart disease was higher in the participants taking the supplement than in those taking the placebo.

For those who only glanced at the headlines or heard the word "ineffective" shouted from a news broadcast, the study results might have seemed to damn beta carotene. In fact, however, what was being damned was not beta carotene, the natural substance, but beta carotene, the "magic" pill, the synthetic supplement. The difference is important. The *real* beta carotene that occurs naturally in both fruits and vegetables is very good for you indeed, especially when it combines with other phytochemicals. The National Cancer Institute confirmed that conclusion.

The Power of This PowerFood

Fruits are loaded with health benefits. To begin with, since water makes up 80 percent to 95 percent of most fruits, they are low in calories. In addition, fruits are excellent sources of fiber, both soluble and insoluble. The insoluble fibers are what determines a fruit's texture—an apple's crunchiness, the mealiness of the papaya, the chewy tang of a citrus fruit—and they have beneficial effects on proper waste elimination. The soluble fibers, especially pectin, are particularly effective in helping to lower cholesterol levels. Fruits are also rich in minerals. Bananas and oranges have high potassium content, while berries supply lots of iron. In addition, most fruits supply boron, a mineral vitally important to bone strength. Above all, fruits are treasure-houses of vitamins, particularly of Vitamin C. The citrus fruits, berries, melons, tropical fruits, and the yellows and oranges—apricots, peaches, nectarines, mangoes—are particularly good Vitamin C sources.

To all this must now be added the evidence that current research is yielding about the phytochemical power in the red, yellow, and orange fruits. Beta carotene, for all its newsworthiness, is only one of the 600-plus carotenoids that have thus far been identified by scientists. Carotenoids are serious antioxidants, but that is not all they do. Scientists believe they invigorate the communication among healthy cells, thus keeping cancer cells from gaining the upper hand.

The red, yellow, and orange fruits are also rich in flavonoids, of which some 800 have been identified to date. Flavonoids function as antioxidants that block carcinogens. They also suppress malignant changes, appear to interfere with hormone-binding to inhibit cancer development, and even help keep collagen healthy. Collagen is the intercellular cement that gives tissue its structure; it's what keeps our skin from wrinkling and our bones from crumbling.

Quercetin is one of the most powerful of the flavonoids, and it adds to its cancer-fighting properties some particularly potent capabilities for protecting the eyes. A number of studies have now identified quercetin, in combination with other carotenoids, as a key weapon against both cataracts and macular degeneration. Quercetin also appears to play a part in blocking the oxidants that lead to respiratory diseases, especially asthma.

How much disease-fighting, anti-aging power is there in this phytochemical group? The Agricultural Research Service of the U.S. Department of Agriculture provides lists of the chemical constituents of various PowerFoods. The USDA's analysis of the chemical power in the melon uses many terms to describe rutin, one of the major flavonoid substances in red, yellow, and orange fruits, including "anti-capillary-fragility; antitumor-promotor; antiapoplectic; anticataract; anticonvulsant; antidiabetic; antiherpetic; antihistaminic; antihypertensive; antiinflammatory; antioxidant; antiviral; cancer-preventive."[*] The analysis of an orange reveals that hesperidin, another of the key flavonoids, is "antiallergenic; antiflu; anti-inflammatory; antioxidant; antivaccinia; antiviral; capillariprotective."[†] And here's what the USDA says about quercetin: "antitumor-promotor; antiasthmatic; anticarcinogenic; antiplaque; cancer-preventive; capillariprotective."[‡]

The flavonoids can be said to be cellular bodyguards; they work as sentries against the entire spectrum of illness known to us. They stand

<hr />

[*]Beckstrom-Sternberg, Stephen M. and Duke, James A. Phytochemeco Database-USDA-ARS-NGRL, Farmacy Query, Microsoft Internet Explorer.
[†]*Ibid.*
[‡]*Ibid.*

on duty outside our cells, keeping disease at bay. That's a lot of disease-prevention and resistance to aging every time you have a breakfast orange, or snack on an apple in mid-afternoon, or pop some grapes into your mouth after dinner. Or even drink a glass of wine.

Other powerful phytochemicals in this group of PowerFoods include:

○ **Ellagic acids, which are found especially in strawberries, grapes, raspberries, and apples. They help neutralize the carcinogens that are particular to contemporary life— the carcinogens in tobacco smoke, processed food, barbecued meats**

○ **Phenols, which inhibit the formation of nitrosamines, thus helping to resist cancer**

○ **Terpenes, credited by researchers with interfering with carcinogenic action**

Clinical trials confirm the effectiveness of this PowerFood. One study in Switzerland, for example, found that women who ate the most fruits, particularly oranges, had half the risk of uterine cancer of women who ate the least. A number of studies provide evidence that diets rich in fruits can stave off heart attacks and even cut down on stroke damage through the artery-unclogging that the fruits seem to stimulate. The red, yellow, and orange fruits are also effective against high blood pressure; in an experiment in Italy, 81 percent of hypertensive patients who ate three to six servings a day were able to halve their daily medication, and some went off the drugs altogether. During the 1970s and eighties, a number of studies yielded evidence that this PowerFood fights viruses like herpes simplex and bacterial growth, and that it helps strengthen the blood capillaries while fighting off cell deterioration.

It is not surprising that researchers, dietitians, and the government advise us to eat five helpings of fruit and vegetables a day; in the case of fruit, a helping means any medium-sized single item—an apple, an orange, a bunch of grapes. As with all PowerFoods, the benefits are especially potent when you eat more than one kind of fruit. Fortunately, the variety of these fruits is so extensive that, singly or in combination, they offer something for every taste and every mood. Red, yellow, and orange fruits are delicious, sweet, life-giving, and packed with power to do us good.

Buying, Handling, and Serving Red, Yellow, and Orange Fruits

Fruits should of course be eaten when ripe, after the enzymatic changes that achieve the fruit's final maturing have been completed. That's when the fruit is at full nutritive power and has realized all it can in taste and aroma. In North America, fruits are harvested in the summer season. The fact is, however, that we live in a global village and can shop in a global marketplace. When it is winter in our part of the world, it is summer south of the equator, and fresh fruits and vegetables from below the border routinely find their way to markets in every region of North America. In effect, fresh fruits and vegetables are available all year round.

Some fruits that must travel considerable distances to market, however, are harvested before the enzymatic process has finished so that the ripening can continue during the journey. Green bananas and peaches will finish ripening just fine on your windowsill. Fruits such as berries and apples stop ripening the minute they're picked, however, and are often treated with ethylene gas and/or kept in cold storage for the journey from farm to the market. Keep that in mind when you buy.

Mostly, buying fruit is a matter of common sense. You want undamaged, "healthy-looking" samples that smell good (or don't smell at all). Much of the fruit that is sold year-round is canned or frozen. Generally, frozen fruits have been chilled without any cooking process; this means they still have most, if not all, of their nutrients. Where canned fruits were once processed to the extent that much of their nutrient power was destroyed, new canning methods have made a dramatic difference in preserving more of the important nutrients and phytochemicals. If you do buy canned fruit, be sure to get it packed in water or unsweetened juice. The heavy syrups in which so many fruits are packed are both calorie-heavy and superfluous—why would you *add* sweetener to fruit?

The best way to eat this PowerFood is fresh—unpeeled, if the skin is edible. (When eating unpeeled fruit, be sure to wash the fruit well to remove any pesticide residue.) Fresh fruit is delicious combined with other fruits, served in salads, as side dishes, as a garnish for meats and poultry, as an accompaniment to dairy products like yogurt, and eaten alone as a quick snack. Kathie Swift, Director of Nutrition at Canyon Ranch in the Berkshires, a highly trained nutrition scientist and a registered dietitian, recommends red, yellow, and orange fruits—as opposed to bagels, rice cakes, or pretzels—as the perfect pick-me-up snack for that low time in the afternoon. Many fruits are also wonderful when cooked—baked, grilled, or poached. There are also fruit compotes and fruit shakes (what we might call processed fresh fruits) that taste sensational and offer, in an altered state, equivalent phytochemical strength.

Fruit spreads are a wonderful low-fat alternative to butter, cheese, and margarine. Here's a quick and easy way to get more fresh fruit into your homemade fruit spreads without added sugar, without pectin, without mason jars, without paraffin, without a lot of trouble. You want fresh, ripe fruits or berries—anything from the ordinary apricot, for example, to the more exotic quince, currants, and gooseberries. Cook the fresh fruit in a small amount of water, just enough to keep it from sticking to the pot, until it's tender. Add an equal amount of a commercial jam or jelly of your choice. Heat the mixture until the fresh fruit and the jam or jelly are thoroughly integrated. Then just repackage the blend in small portions and keep them in the freezer, not the refrigerator. This process reduces the sugar content of the commercial jam or jelly by half, and it adds the nutrients and phytochemical benefits of the fresh fruit—the best of both worlds. Some of my particular favorites are: fresh apricots combined with store-bought ginger marmalade; fresh rhubarb with strawberry jam; and fresh red currants with red currant jelly.

The number of red, yellow, and orange fruits is considerable, their variety is wide-ranging, and the possibilities for different uses are almost limitless. Here are some hints on just a few of my favorites, a small but representative cross section of these PowerFoods:

PowerFoods

Apricots

The apricot is a powerhouse of beta carotene and the other carotenoids. Diets rich in apricots appear to offer some protection against cancers of the mouth, throat, esophagus, stomach, bladder—even the lung.

It was no doubt because of their nutritional wallop that apricots were made a part of the astronauts' diet on a number of NASA missions, including the Apollo moon shots. If the voyage to the moon was this fruit's longest journey, it was not, however, its first; apricots originated in China, spread across Asia into Europe, and were brought to California in the eighteenth century by Spaniards. California has since become a major grower of apricots.

Fresh or dried, the apricot is golden orange in color. At full ripeness, it feels slightly soft. The ripe fruits will last three to five days in the refrigerator. Combine apricots with raspberries, or with dried figs and prunes, or with almonds for a superior taste treat.

Bananas

This is the quintessential yellow fruit, although you can easily buy a bunch that is quite green, then watch it ripen in a day or two. Bananas are ripe when the peel is solid yellow. Never refrigerate bananas; it turns them black.

Bananas grow on what looks like a tree but is actually an aboveground stem. The stem is made up of leafstalks growing one inside the other; these are the banana bunches.

In addition to their power, bananas are unmatched for convenience. Stick one in the lunchbox, the briefcase, the backpack. Best of all, you don't need to bag them or wrap them in plastic; they come in their own ready-made packages.

Cantaloupe and Other Melons

The cantaloupe, really a muskmelon, is the most popular melon in the United States, although it comes originally from Europe. The fragrant orange flesh, protected by its tan rind, is a dead giveaway to cantaloupe's high carotene content; the same goes for the casaba, the Crenshaw, and the watermelon. The latter is particularly rich in the phytochemicals that fight cancer of the esophagus.

Once harvested, melons become softer. Since the only way to tell ripeness for certain is by cutting the melon open, which stores naturally will not allow, it's important to take some care in choosing the melon you'll take home. At the melon bin you see the ritual sniffers and hoisters. In this case, do as they do.

Sniff for fragrance, which indicates ripeness. A lack of fragrance does not mean the melon is bad, although a smell of decay or rottenness certainly does; rather, the lack of fragrance may mean you'll have to keep the melon around a day or two before it hits its sweetness peak. Melons differ in shape, but any melon you buy should have a full, regular, symmetrical shape, whether it's round like a cantaloupe or Crenshaw, or oval like a watermelon.

Check out the rind. A cantaloupe should have even, gray netting with little or no trace of green. It should feel slightly soft, but not spongy; a hard, green cantaloupe is not a good buy. Casabas and Crenshaws should have yellow rinds, and both should feel a little springy at the ends. Watermelons should be deep green in color and neither wax-shiny nor dingy dull. Check the underside, the part that rested on the ground during growing: It should be pale yellow; if the underbelly is greenish or white, that indicates that the melon was picked early and will lack sweetness. Check the stem, if any remains: If it is green, the melon was picked too soon, if dry and brown, the melon is ripe and ready.

Melons bought a bit firm should stay at room temperature for a day or two to soften. Ripe melons are best stored in the refrigerator.

Grapes

Even though there are green grapes, the red and purple varieties qualify grapes as belonging to the red, yellow, and orange fruits. (The green grapes are good for you, but they lack lycopene, and the health benefits that the red pigment lycopene imparts.) Grapes are the "fruit of the vine," as the Old Testament puts it, cultivated since time immemorial to be served as a fresh fruit, as dried raisins, as a preserved jelly, or crushed and fermented as wine. And from time immemorial, grapes have been thought to possess healing power, even if it was the healing of heightened sensation and reduced pain achieved through inebriation. More recently, the so-called "grape cure" was a favorite of natural health advocates, said to be efficacious against cancer. Today, as with so many of the cures put forward by health faddists and vegetable-diet "cranks," science confirms that a range of phytochemicals in grapes makes them a particularly effective disease-fighter. Specifically, the high level of ellagic acid in grapes is effective in resisting and neutralizing the cancers that result directly from so many of the pollutants of our era: tobacco smoke, processed foods, barbecued meats.

Grapes come in any number of varieties available in the markets today, although all descend from two basic types—the European, thought to have been brought to California by Spanish missionaries in the eighteenth century, and the American, the native species growing along the northeastern coast, among other locations, that prompted explorer Leif Eriksson to give the name "Vineland" to the North American continent he had stumbled upon. Both types of grape are cultivated on the North American continent today, although the European types predominate. The native American varieties—like Concord and Catawba—are grown mostly in the eastern U.S. and are harvested in the fall. The numerous European varieties are grown mostly in California. Red grapes are halfway in color between the pale green of Thompson Seedless, for example, and the dusky purple of Concords or Exotics. Some common varieties are Flame Seedless, Red Globe, Ruby Seedless, Exotic, Black Beauty, Ribier, and Champagne.

Grapes are easy to select: buy plump, clean-looking bunches that are firmly attached to pliable green stems. Rinse the grapes under water, and store them in the refrigerator where they will keep for about a week.

If I were forced to make a choice, I would have to say that grapes are my all-time favorite fruit (when fresh figs are not available). I always keep a bunch on hand and love to alternate among the almost endless variety. I eat grapes whole—skins as well as pulp, chewing the seeds and then swallowing them. In fact, grape skins and seeds are chock-full of phytochemical richness, so if you can manage to chew them, you should.

Kumquats

This Chinese word means gold orange. The kumquat is the smallest of the citrus fruits, as decorative as it is delicious and as nutritious as it is decorative. Its intense orange color indicates an intense presence of carotenoids. Kumquats offer flavonoids and phenols as well.

The great thing about the kumquat is that, unlike other citrus fruits, you eat the whole thing—the thin, sweet rind as well as the golden orange, pungent flesh. Keep that in mind when you shop for kumquats; look for plump, shiny fruits with an even, deep color and a smooth, unbruised skin. Kumquats are sold mostly in the wintertime and are now routinely found in well-stocked supermarkets.

To eat them, pinch the fruit between your fingers first; this sets the juices flowing and mingles the tartness of the flesh with the sweetness of the skin.

Mango

The fruit of an evergreen tree of the sumac family, the mango is native to tropical Asia and is symbolic of South Sea islands and equatorial lushness. Its yellow orange flesh is thick with carotenoids; in fact, mangoes offer more beta carotene than carotene-rich apricots and cantaloupe.

When shopping for mangoes, look for a skin of deep green shading to bright yellow and red. A freckled appearance is common. The ripe fruit yields to slight pressure and has a distinctive fragrance; beware even a whiff of fermentation. In the refrigerator, mangoes can last for two weeks, but leave underripe fruits at room temperature to soften for a few days first.

What tends to keep people from eating mangoes is not so much their unfamiliarity—they are becoming a fairly standard offering— but the perceived difficulty in eating them. The problem is the tenacious hold the flesh has on the pit. One way around this is just to peel the mango and eat it right down to the stone as you would a peach. Peeling presents its own difficulties, however: The juicy fruit is slippery and hard to handle. A better idea is to wet the skin thoroughly, then cut the fruit lengthwise away from the pit (in slices if necessary), then peel the skin off as if the mango were a banana, or pare it off with a vegetable parer. Another way is a variation on the hiker's method of eating an orange. Roll the mango on a tabletop (or on a rock or the ground, if you're out hiking) until the flesh inside feels soft. Then cut a square hole in the stem end and suck out the juice and then the pulp. It may not be pretty, but it's effective.

Sprinkle some lime juice on sliced mango for a particularly refreshing dessert or snack.

(Caution: Just as some members of the sumac family produce a toxin to which people are highly allergic, the mango *skin* contains a chemical that produces a rash on contact; unfortunately, this hyper-sensitivity is fairly common, so while you can certainly enjoy the pulp, exercise caution with the skin.)

Nectarines

Like apricots—and peaches, plums, and cherries—nectarines are drupes, typically fleshy fruits with a single hard stone enclosing the seed. Some think of the nectarine as a peach without fuzz. It can be used in the same ways as a peach, and, like peaches, nectarines can be canned or frozen. But nectarines, more so than peaches, are rich in the carotenoids and flavonoids that serve as antioxidants, that improve the body's uptake of protein, and that fight degeneration and bolster immunity. It is no accident that this PowerFood was named for nec-tar—in ancient Greek myth, the fruit of the gods.

Nectarines are a deep yellow with a reddish blush. When buying, look for well-rounded specimens with a slight "give." Harder fruits will take a couple of days to ripen, but make sure you do not get greenish specimens; they were simply picked too soon, and they won't ripen at all. The give in the surface means the fruits are ready to eat; they will stay fresh in the refrigerator for another four days or so.

Nectarines are wonderful when baked, grilled, or poached. They are a superb breakfast, alone or as an accompaniment to cereal and milk or yogurt. Blend a nectarine and an orange for a great shake. Nectarines go particularly well with meat or poultry. Try slices of baked or grilled nectarines with ham or use them as a garnish the next time you barbecue a chicken.

Papaya

The papaya, also known as the pawpaw, is another treat that smacks of the tropics. In fact, some historians believe it is native to the Caribbean islands, although most of today's domestic crop comes from Hawaii. Papayas offer considerable phytochemical power, great taste, and versatility.

The golden orange flesh of this fruit, lightly tinged with pink, is an indication of its carotenoid content. It also contains flavonoids, protease inhibitors that keep viruses in check, and an enzyme that aids digestion.

In shopping for papaya, look for skin that is green tinged with rose and a creamy yellow orange. The shape should be pearlike, but the papaya is much larger than a pear. Sniff the stem end; the ripe papaya should have a sweet fragrance, never harsh. In the refrigerator, papaya lasts about a week.

To eat, peel the fruit, then scoop out the black seeds and save them. In sharp contrast to the sugar-sweet taste of the papaya flesh, the seeds are pepper-hot and crunchy. They make an unusual, caperlike garnish, or grind them in a food processor and use as a peppery seasoning. Use the papaya flesh in fruit salad, shakes, puréed as a sauce for poultry, as a garnish on fish, or as an accompaniment to just about anything you might barbecue. A woman I know, traveling in Hawaii, started her morning with cereal and milk in the half-shell of a papaya, then used the other half as the serving bowl for her tuna salad lunch, and at dinner used two halves of yet another papaya, one half for the crab salad main course, one for the dessert of sherbet and cut-up fresh fruit.

Pineapple

Another yellow fruit, the pineapple is tropical and grows in small bunches around a stalk. When pineapple is processed for canning, every part of it is used. The flesh is sliced and cut into chunks. The inside of the shell is scraped for crushed pineapple. The trimmings are shredded and dried to make pineapple bran for livestock. The enzyme bromelin, which can be extracted from the flesh during the processing, is used in meat-tenderizing and as a flavor enhancer.

Fresh pineapple is 85 percent water. Its remaining 15 percent packs a phytochemical wallop over and above its other nutrients—specifically, Vitamin C and manganese. Pineapple's phytochemical collection includes carotenoids and flavonoids. It also contains the bromelin enzyme, which helps prevent blood clots from forming.

Pineapple will not ripen after it is picked, so what you buy is what you get. A good test for ripeness is to smell the base of the fruit; it should smell sweet. The pineapple should not be too green in color, and although it should be firm to the touch, there should be some "give."

Store uncut pineapple at room temperature. If you want it to be at its maximum sweetness, turn it upside down, prop it up against something (like the kitchen wall), and leave it overnight. This lets the sugars in the bottom move through the length of the fruit.

Pineapple's pungent sweetness makes it excellent in salads and stuffings, in breakfast cereals and dessert, grilled on skewers with poultry or seafood, basted with orange or lemon juice, or with cloves or ginger—as well as all by itself.

Raspberries and Strawberries

Raspberries and strawberries are among the sweetest of the PowerFoods—and the most powerful, particularly rich in cancer-fighting ellagic acids as well as in lycopene.

They are best bought when they are in season and locally grown wherever you live. They should be stout and firm. If you are buying them in a box, make sure that the top layer of fruit looks good and that the box itself is not stained or damp. When buying from a bin, be sure the color is uniform, and avoid crushed or withered berries. The caps of strawberries should be bright green.

Because of their delicacy, raspberries should be handled with great care. Don't, for example, wash them in a strong spurt of water; it could crush them. Be gentle as you rinse the berries and pat them dry. The fragility of raspberries also means they must be eaten as soon as possible after being picked. Eat fresh raspberries within 24 hours of purchase. Strawberries are only slightly tougher than raspberries; eat them within two days of purchase.

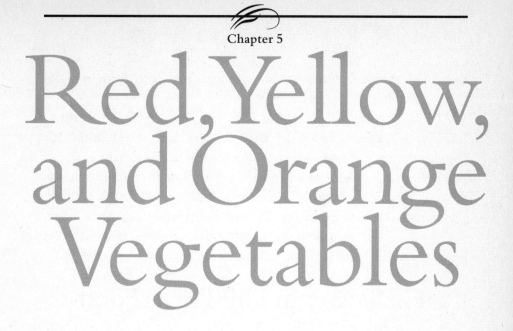

Chapter 5

Red, Yellow, and Orange Vegetables

*Several carefully studied populations in Mediterranean
countries and in some areas in Asia where traditional diets consist
largely of foods of plant origin exhibit long life expectancies and low
rates of many chronic diseases. Studies provide further evidence
that high consumption of vegetables confers numerous health benefits.
The carotenoids, as well as the vitamins, minerals, and fiber that
are abundant in the plant-based diet appear to play important roles
in the prevention of several cancers, coronanry heart disease, neural
tube defects, and cataracts.*

—WALTER C. WILLETT, M.D., DR. P. H.
HARVARD SCHOOL OF PUBLIC HEALTH

*t*raditionally, the American way of
eating has put vegetables second to meat—an accompaniment
amounting to perhaps two servings a day, on average. There are some
indications that that may be changing now. Americans have become
more adventurous eaters, and in response, farmers have extended the
range of vegetables they plant and harvest. Part of the reason may be

that medical and scientific authorities have begun to recommend a plant-based diet for optimal health.

The versatility of red, yellow, and orange vegetables—tomatoes, beets, squash, carrots, red and yellow peppers, and sweet potatoes, to name the most popular—makes them ideally suited to take pride of place in main courses, or to replace meat altogether. Consider the tomato's range of uses in chili, salsa, and all manner of sauces. Carrots, the eternal side dish, make terrific and filling salads as well as soups. Sweet potatoes are decadent snacks when prepared as chips, and sweet potato pancakes are a meal unto themselves.

The Power in This PowerFood

Like the fruits with which they share pigments, the red, yellow, and orange vegetables are rich in carotenoids and flavonoids. The vegetables, however, offer different combinations of these and other phytochemicals as well as different fiber, vitamin, and mineral content, and different textures, tastes, and uses.

Carotenoids derive their name from the fact that they share orange pigment with carrots. Not just carrots but all the red, yellow, and orange vegetables are loaded with the carotenoids—especially beta carotene and lycopene. In the face of the beta carotene controversy discussed in the previous chapter, new research today is demonstrating that carotenoids other than beta carotene may have just as much antioxidant power as beta carotene. In fact, these studies show that many other vegetable carotenoids block carcinogens and prevent cells in test tubes from becoming malignant.

In other words, it looks as if it's the carotenoid cocktail that packs the wallop, not just a particular carotenoid and certainly not just one substance in isolation. In other words, it's better to eat the whole carrot, and it's better still to eat it in combination with tomatoes and sweet potatoes or other PowerFoods.

To date, over 600 carotenoids have been identified. As antioxidants, the carotenoids also protect heart health, act as anti-inflammatories, and help us resist the effects of aging. The antioxidant power of the red, yellow, and orange vegetables, combined with their heavy doses of

Vitamins C and E and intense concentrations of both soluble and insoluble fibers, make these PowerFoods exceptional fighters against degenerative diseases.

Buying, Storing, and Preparing the Red, Yellow, and Orange Vegetables

These PowerFoods include roots (beets and carrots), gourds (squash), and one vegetable that is really a fruit (tomato), so their care and handling differs from food to food. (Yes, the tomato *is* a fruit, but it is eaten as a vegetable. You would not eat a tomato for dessert, for example, as you would a fruit. And on a pizza, you would certainly rather have tomato sauce than fruit sauce.)

Beets

Roots whose greens are also edible (see Chapter 6, Cruciferous and Leafy Green Vegetables), beets taste just about as sweet as sugar. In fact, when Napoleon's ships blockaded Europe in the nineteenth century, preventing regular sugar cane shipments, a commercial sweetener was produced from beets, and beet production soared.

Long before Napoleon, however, in fact since ancient times, beets were thought of as helpful for all sorts of gastrointestinal disorders and as an anti-inflammatory pain-fighter. Today, we know that beets may indeed be rejuvenative for just about every bodily organ and every body system. Heavy concentrations of carotenoids and flavonoids work as antioxidants to reduce the accumulation of plaque in arteries and promote cell differentiation, thus acting as a powerful anticancer agent, while other phytochemicals work to cleanse the blood and nourish the circulation.

When buying beets, be aware of the general rule of thumb that the smaller the beet, the more tender it is likely to be. Very small baby beets, found early in the summer, are a true delicacy. If you're buying a bunch of beets, they should be fairly uniform in size, so that they will cook evenly. If buying beets with their greens, keep in mind that the greens deteriorate before the root does, so a slight wilting of greens does not necessarily mean bad roots as long as the beet root is still firm. With the greens removed, beets last at least three weeks in the refrigerator. Canned beets lack some of the nutritive power of fresh beets, and much of their taste and texture, but they are an acceptable substitute.

Scrub the beets gently before cooking, taking care not to break the skin. Beets can be baked, boiled, microwaved, or steamed. Do not cut or peel them before cooking them in liquid; rather, wait until they have cooled, when the skins will easily slip off.

Beets are ideal in salad and soups. The classic beet soup borscht is served hot with spices in winter or cold and sweet in summer, often garnished with plain yogurt or sour cream. Sprinkle grated beets over potatoes or other cooked vegetables, or use to "sweeten" grated horseradish to mellow its sting.

Carrots

The ancient Greeks fed carrots to their horses to improve the animals' respiration; they also prescribed carrot juice for indigestion and skin problems, and they drank it when they wanted an aphrodisiac. Current research confirms the efficacy of carrots as a defense against respiratory ills and as a cholesterol reducer—and they may indeed supply a compound that stimulates the sexual appetite.

Fresh carrots are available all year round, coming to a supermarket near you most probably from Michigan or California, or available from local farm stands in season. You can typically find baby carrots as well as "adult" carrots; the baby carrots have been picked early and are particularly tender, although they lack the sweet taste of the larger vegetables, which contain more sugar than most other vegetables. Look for smooth carrots, with a beautiful orange color and fresh bright greens sprouting from the top. Carrots also come frozen and canned, but since fresh carrots are available all year round, neither the frozen nor the canned variety is worth buying.

Store carrots in plastic in the refrigerator. Away from apples or pears, which tend to pass along the bitterness of escaping ethylene gas; the carrots should last two to three weeks. Scrub the carrots well before eating, and, if you like, peel off the skin. While many vegetables lose nutrients when cooked, the opposite is true with carrots. Cooking almost doubles the availability of carotenoids and other phytochemicals. Cook the carrots—bake, blanch, microwave, or steam them—until they are just tender-crisp; overcooking reduces all available nutrients.

Chopped or grated carrots add taste and texture to pasta, stir-fries, stews, soups, platters of cooked vegetables, potato pancakes, muffins, and breads, as well as to carrot cake. The latter, however, is highly caloric, with a very high fat content; substitute apple sauce for oil, and you cut the fat content considerably. One of my favorite quick-and-easy carrot snacks is simply to grate two carrots, combine with one tablespoon of raisins, squeeze on a little lemon juice, spray on a drizzle of olive oil, add salt and pepper to taste.

Squash

More than forty kinds of gourd-shaped vegetables qualify as squash, including many plants we tend to refer to as pumpkins. They are as genuinely American as anything you can find. Indigenous to this hemisphere, squash plants sustained Native Americans for at least five thousand years before the coming of European colonists, who quickly made the squash a mainstay of their diet once local tribes taught them how to harvest and prepare it. The word "squash" comes from "askutasquash," a native American word meaning "something eaten raw." But Native Americans knew lots of ways to cook squash, too.

Squashes grow on bushes or vines, have five-pointed leaves and yellow orange flowers, and come in numerous colors, sizes, shapes, and tastes. Squash flowers can also be eaten, but it is the vegetable portion that most of us eat, and it is there that so much nutrition is found.

There are two major groups of squash, summer and winter. Summer squashes grown on bushes and tend to be yellow or green (like yellow crookneck and zucchini) and the tint of their flesh is somewhat pale. Because the fruits are picked when still immature, with a soft rind, and because these squashes are more than 95 percent water, they offer only moderate nutritive value.

Summer squashes should be eaten as soon as possible after harvesting. The taste of these squashes is subtle, making them a good accompaniment to more assertive flavors. Eat them raw, steamed, stir-fried, or stuffed and baked. Add them to salads, casseroles, soups, and pasta dishes. Grated, they make wonderful pancakes, not to mention dessert cakes.

Certainly, summer squashes are low in fat and sodium, delicious, and good for you in the way all fruits and vegetables are good for you, but when it comes to packing the real disease-fighting punch, the PowerFood to reckon with is winter squash.

There is a great variety of winter squash—acorn, buttercup (my favorite), butternut, calabaza, Hubbard, pumpkin, and more. These squashes keep for months when stored in a cool, dry place. *Dry* is the key word here; any hint of dampness in the storage area, and the squash will rot. But kept dry, the squashes you buy in late autumn should last the whole winter, which is what makes squash so reliable and convenient.

All squashes should be firm and unblemished. Take care that the delicate skin of the summer squashes has not been pierced by a shopper testing for freshness; once it is punctured, the flesh will begin to decay.

The winter squashes offer a darker flesh and a wider variety of tastes and textures than the summer squashes. Winter squashes are almost all eaten cooked. They are wonderful baked, boiled, microwaved, sautéed, and steamed.

Winter squashes can be cut in half and baked in the rind until tender (remove seeds and stringy pulp first). Sprinkle each half with spices if you're in the mood for something savory, or top with syrup or honey if you prefer it sweet. Alternatively, the baked half can be the receptacle for a variety of fillings—rice, meat, vegetables.

Winter squashes lend themselves to more dishes when they are peeled, cubed, and then steamed, blanched, sautéed, or even stir-fried. The cooked flesh can then be puréed for use in soups and stews or as a filling. What kind of filling? Think Thanksgiving, and pumpkin pie.

Here's something I do whenever I blanch, boil, or steam winter squash. After cooking, I drain the cooking water, add some fresh water to make up for evaporative losses, and freeze it to use the next time I blanch, boil, or steam winter squash. This way, you never lose any flavor, which, for people who love squash as much as I do, is certainly a good thing. In addition, there is a buildup of squash flavor in the cooking water, time after time, so that by the end of the squash season, I have a squash stock that can be the beginning of a delicious soup.

Another favorite quick and easy trick with squash is to scoop out the cooked flesh, mash it with a little cinnamon, nutmeg, salt and pepper, add canned crushed pineapple, mandarin orange segments, or applesauce, and a little squash cooking water for consistency. It makes a great side-dish casserole, delicious enough for your best company.

While all the squashes contribute to heart health, it is these winter squashes with their deep orange flesh that can be such a knockout punch against cancers of the esophagus, stomach, lung, bladder, larynx, and prostate. Researchers in both Japan and the U.S., in fact, have found that a high intake of squash can prevent and control lung cancer even among heavy smokers; it also serves as protection against secondhand smoke.

While the seeds of most winter squashes are typically discarded, those of the pumpkin have been shown to be rich in protease inhibitors that fight intestinal viruses and reproductive dysfunctions. The pumpkin seed oil, meanwhile, seems to go after the free radicals that are responsible for arthritis, and for arthritis pain. Perhaps the Zuni of Arizona knew what they were doing when they used pumpkin seeds and squash flowers to heal wounds and scars. There is certainly healing power in these PowerFoods.

Sweet Potato

The sweet potato is neither a potato nor a yam. Instead, the sweet potato belongs to the morning glory family, and it is one of the most nutritious of the PowerFoods.

A native of the New World, the sweet potato was brought back east to Europe by Columbus and was later widely cultivated by colonials. It was also carried west from the Americas—surely from the coast of South America—most probably by the ancient Polynesian sea voyagers who, in their sailing canoes, populated so many of the islands of the South Seas, where the sweet potato remains a staple food today.

This important tropical root crop is loaded with high concentrations of antioxidant carotenoids, flavonoids, and phenolic acids. That makes the sweet potato a powerful fighter against such diseases as uterine and lung cancers. As with the richly colored squashes, sweet potato has been shown to be particularly effective against the dangers of cigarette smoke—your own or someone else's.

Hunt for sweet potatoes that feel heavy in the hand. Avoid any that are bruised or that have blackened areas. The color of sweet potato skin can range from a light toast color to a burnished red; whatever the hue, the color should be clear. In a cool place—but never in the refrigerator, where sugars turn to starch—sweet potatoes can last for up to two months. Brush off excess dirt before storing sweet potatoes, but don't wash them until you're ready to cook them. Handle sweet potatoes with care; the skin is delicate.

The natural sweetness of sweet potatoes intensifies during storage and is further augmented by cooking. For that reason—and possibly because a popular Thanksgiving preparation has them covered with marshmallows—people tend to think that sweet potatoes are fattening. It ain't necessarily so. Sweet potato and white potato are about equal calorically, and neither contains fat. In fact, precisely because of its rich flavor, if you substitute a sweet potato for a white potato in a recipe, you can probably cut back on the quantities of butter or sugar the recipe calls for.

Sweet potatoes are delicious baked, although they can also be simmered, steamed, or microwaved. My baking method starts with scrubbing and rinsing the sweet potato, but not drying it. Pierce the skin in several places with a fork, wrap it loosely in aluminum foil, and bake it for one and a half to two hours at 400° F. on the lowest oven rack. Yum! Soft, sweet, it needs no enhancement; I eat it as is. What's more, as nutritionist Kathie Swift reminds us, cooked sweet potatoes are delicious cold. She recommends packing one for lunch or for an afternoon snack, tossing in an orange or papaya for accompaniment.

Many people eat sweet potatoes only at Thanksgiving, and that's a pity. Their texture and taste make them a fragrant and tasty element of a variety of dishes—in soups and stews, as a match for chicken, and, as you'll see in the recipes, even as potato chips!

PowerFoods

Tomatoes

Although the U.S. Supreme Court declared the tomato a vegetable in 1893 (for tariff and customs purposes), it is in fact a fruit. Actually, it's a berry, a member of the nightshade family, and, like its cousin, the deadly nightshade, was for centuries considered a poisonous plant. The Spanish conquistadors found the tomato in South America in the 1500s and brought it back to Europe, where it decorated gardens but was only eaten, if at all, after it had been cooked for hours. The Italians did not get hold of the tomato until 1522; they have certainly done a lot with it since then.

In the U.S., one legend has it that a young scientist offered to prove that tomatoes were nontoxic by eating one in public, onstage, at the New Jersey State Fair in the early years of the twentieth century. Since his successful exhibition, the tomato has become a major crop of New Jersey's truck farms. Most year-round tomatoes, however, are grown in California and Florida and have been bred for toughness to survive their wintertime journeys to the supermarkets of the rest of the country. As a result, they are tasteless. I eat tomatoes only in summer, right off the vine in my garden or from the local farm stand.

The rest of the year, it's a good idea to eat tomatoes canned; in doing so, we may well lower our chances of getting cancer. That, at least, is what several tracking studies show. Northern Italians, the famous tomato-eaters mentioned earlier, evidence 60 percent lower risk of cancers of the mouth, esophagus, stomach, colon, and rectum. Low rates of stomach cancer are found among tomato-happy Hawaiians. There is reduced incidence of lung cancer among Norwegians, who eat a lot of tomatoes, and reduced risk of prostate cancer among Americans who eat lots of tomatoes versus those who eat few or none. A five-year survey performed by the Harvard Medical School found that the chances of dying of any kind of cancer were lowest among people who ate tomatoes (or strawberries) weekly.

Much of the tomato's cancer-fighting prowess is attributable to the carotenoid lycopene, provider of its red pigment. Almost as potent are the coumarins and phenolic acids that block that notorious carcinogen, nitrosamine, which might otherwise be formed in the body.

Tomatoes are also, of course, rich in Vitamins A and C; they contain some fiber; they offer minerals, especially potassium; and they weigh in at about 30 calories per tomato.

When shopping for tomatoes, from cherry tomatoes to the beefsteaks, look for smooth, plump, fragrant specimens. Do not buy them from a refrigerated case, and never refrigerate less than ripe tomatoes once you get them home; cold retards the ripening process. Less than ripe tomatoes will ripen at home in due course. If you place them on a windowsill in the sun, they will ripen fast, but probably unevenly, and they will certainly lose flavor. A better method is to place them in a paper bag with a ripe apple or banana. The ethylene gas that such fruits naturally emit will ripen the tomatoes quickly.

Tomatoes can be baked, broiled, sautéed, or stewed. To peel them, blanch in boiling water for 30 seconds, then quickly rinse them in cold water. The skin will peel off easily with a paring knife.

Sautéed with garlic and spices, stuffed with grains and nuts and then baked, or layered and baked, with some olive oil sprinkled over them, tomatoes can easily be the centerpiece of any meal. Of course, they are wonderful as a side dish anytime, and chopped tomatoes combine with all manner of other condiments to make salsa or pasta sauce. As to raw tomatoes for salads, wait for summer, and get them locally.

Chapter 6

Cruciferous and Leafy Green Vegetables

Phytochemicals in crucifers and leafy green vegetables appear to trigger increased production of special enzymes in the body's cells that ward off cancer-causing agents. The wisdom of the advice to eat cruciferous vegetables appears stronger than ever.

—DR. PAUL TALALAY,
JOHNS HOPKINS UNIVERSITY SCHOOL OF MEDICINE

*t*raditionally considered "mere" salads and side dishes, the crucifers and leafy greens can easily be moved to the center of a meal. Let's get the terms straight right away:

Some cruciferous vegetables are both leafy and green—kale and collards for example. But not all leafy green vegetables are crucifers; lettuces, for example, are not cruciferous. The word "crucifer" means "cross-bearer," and the *cruciferae,* as the scientific Latin calls them, bear cross-shaped flowers—four petals arranged diagonally. These vegetables are part of the mustard family. They include arugula, bok choy, broccoli, broccoli rabe, brussels sprouts, cabbage, cauliflower, collards, horseradish, kale, kohlrabi, mustard greens, radishes, rutabaga, turnips, and watercress. In recent years, these vegetables have been the subject of wide-ranging research into their considerable and very evident disease-prevention properties.

Just as important as the crucifers, however, in terms of both healing and food planning, are the leafy green vegetables—lettuces, spinach, parsley, endive—about which we should say the greener the better, at least as far as fighting disease is concerned.

Both cruciferous vegetables and leafy greens have high nutrient density. That means they have a high proportion of nutrition—fiber, vitamins, minerals, and carbohydrates—for the few calories supplied. The diversity of these vegetables enhances their health merit. To almost all of the twenty-plus vegetables listed above, add variations on the theme; of the lettuces, for example, no fewer than eighty-seven varieties were listed as far back as 1885 in a U.S. government agricultural report.

The variety—from bland cauliflower to tart mustard greens, from chewy turnips to crunchy romaine lettuce—ensures that there is something here for every palate. Combining the crucifers and leafy greens by mixing and matching colors, tastes, and textures only enhances the variety and synergy that are so important to healthy eating.

What's more, advances in agricultural technology now mean that as a group, crucifers and leafy greens are available all year round. This means that you can find some kind of cruciferous and leafy green vegetable just about any day of the week, any week of the year. In addition to the fresh specimens, of course, it is always possible to find many of these vegetables in frozen form.

The Power in This PowerFood

The crucifers and leafy greens are the preeminent cancer-protective PowerFoods. They are rich in the indoles and sulforaphanes that block cancer-causing agents from reaching cells. They are loaded with the flavonoid antioxidants that scavenge the free radicals. And they are filled with the carotenoids that prevent cancer cells from spreading. (Although the yellow pigment of the carotenoids is covered up by the chlorophyll of the green vegetables, the carotenoids are there in force nevertheless, especially lutein, suspected of being the champion cancer-fighting agent of all, and demonstrably effective in reducing the risk of macular degeneration, the cruel and irreversible loss of vision and the single biggest cause of blindness in older people.)

Clinical trials and laboratory analyses in a number of research centers dedicated to food science, medicine, and nutrition have remarked on the "inhibitory effects" the indoles and sulforaphanes have shown on cancer, particularly cancers of the breast and ovaries, as well as on toxins that give rise to cancerous growth. It is these indoles and sulforaphanes in particular that have made broccoli and cabbage rivals for the title of "premier cancerfighter." (Imagine the power you take in when you eat both.) Both these classes of phytochemicals are responsible for giving the crucifers their pungent taste. In fact, scientists believe that the phytochemicals are actually formed when the plants in which they occur are processed—as, for example, by being chewed or cooked. That action unleashes the indoles and sulforaphanes, which work to keep the carcinogens out of the body's cells.

Cabbage is also strong in the flavonoids that stimulate the body to produce enzymes that fight cancer. Its supply of beta carotene (and lycopene, in red cabbage) makes it a powerful fighter against coronary disease and gastrointestinal disorders, especially ulcers.

Broccoli, which is loaded with sulforaphane, antioxidants, and carotenoids, has been shown to protect against cancers of the esophagus, stomach, colon, lung, larynx, prostate, mouth, pharynx, ovaries, breast, and cervix. In fact, as an all-around antiaging, anticancer package of phytochemicals, broccoli probably edges out cabbage just slightly; at least, the National Cancer Institute ranks it first. The American public ranks it first as well. Brought here by Italian immigrants (the Italians first latched onto broccoli in the seventeenth century; they since have perfected its many uses), broccoli is today grown mostly in California, but it is eaten everywhere. Despite the jokes and even the disdain of former President George Bush, broccoli is America's favorite vegetable.

Here's my favorite way of turning America's favorite into a main course: First, boil six waxy—not baking—potatoes. Let them cool, then peel and mash them. Steam one large head of broccoli, with the stem, until it's very tender. Mash it with a fork. Combine the mashed potatoes and the mashed broccoli, add a cup of sautéed onions, a teaspoon of chopped garlic, and salt and pepper to taste. The blend of flavors and its heartiness make this dish a completely satisfying main course, with enough left over for lunch the next day. For added crunch, toss in one or two tablespoons of toasted sesame seeds, a great source of fiber, essential fatty acids, and calcium.

Buying and Preparing Cruciferous and Leafy Green Vegetables

When buying the flower crucifers—broccoli, cabbage, brussels sprouts, and the like—look for firm, compact heads with closed flower buds. Store them unwashed in open plastic bags in the refrigerator crisper; they'll keep for four or five days.

The root crucifers like radishes, rutabaga, and turnips should be smooth and firm, and their greens should be healthy-looking and intact. Separate the greens and store the vegetables in plastic bags in the crisper. They should last a week. Store beet and turnip greens as you would other leafy vegetables, and prepare them similarly.

When buying leafy greens, look for smaller-leaved plants, which tend to have more flavor. The leaves should be a robust green and should be crisp. Unwashed greens last for up to five days when stored in loose plastic bags in the crisper.

Whether you have bought from the supermarket or the roadside stand, you should wash all vegetables thoroughly. Peel vegetables whose wax coatings don't rinse off easily. On leafy vegetables, crucifer or not, pull off the outermost leaves and trim the tops, then be sure to wash the inner leaves thoroughly.

The reason these vegetables are typically stored in bags in the crisper is that light, heat, and air detract from their nutritional value as well as from their taste and texture. Similarly, long soaking can remove important water-soluble vitamins from them. This is why dishes calling for leafy greens are rarely cooked for long and are best prepared just before you are ready to eat them. Steaming and microwaving, which are both fast and use minimal water, are ideal for cooking crucifers and leafy greens.

Some Leaves from the Crucifer Book

Canyon Ranch nutritionist Kathie Swift tells how, having married a man who thought vegetables meant corn or peas, she slowly and steadily introduced him to the crucifers by sneaking them into other foods. "If I was making a fried rice dish," says Kathie, "I would add small amounts of broccoli. On a turkey sandwich, along with lettuce and tomato, I sandwiched in some watercress. In a beef barley soup, I'd toss in some chopped kale. Even my stuffed peppers hosted some cruciferous vegetables in disguise." The legerdemain worked, a tribute to Kathie's persistence and the good taste and versatility of these vegetables.

All the cruciferous vegetables offer phytochemical power similar to that in broccoli and cabbage. That goes for the aristocratic brussels sprout, the humble turnip, and everything in between. And while broccoli, cauliflower, cabbage, brussels sprouts, watercress, and radishes are fairly common foods to the American table, others are only now beginning to move into the mainstream. Crucifers that were once limited to a single region of the country, to ethnic markets, or to health-food stores are becoming widely available, both for their fresh new taste and their health benefits.

Collards

Collard greens, for example, are a typically Southern food. Early nutritionists attributed to collards the good health of poor Southerners whose diets were otherwise insufficient. This member of the cabbage family, with its deep green, paddlelike leaves, is available year-round and is delicious any number of ways, except raw. It is considered good for the liver and a superior blood cleanser.

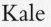

Kale

Kale thrives in the cold; in fact, its flavor is enhanced by frost! For that reason, it is the perfect winter vegetable, especially welcome when other fresh vegetables are hard to come by. No wonder it's so well known in Scotland, from whence Benjamin Franklin brought the first seeds to the United States two centuries ago. Kale has curly leaves, a strong flavor, and a dark green color. In addition to serving as a salad ingredient, kale goes well in stir-fries and is excellent cooked on its own—just squeeze some lemon juice over it. A classic Portuguese dish is kale soup (see the version by our chefs in Part Three).

Broccoli Rabe

Broccoli rabe is considered a delicacy by many and too aggressively pungent by some. The stalk, leaf, and flower of this nonheading variety of broccoli are all edible, and all add zest to bland dishes. They also add vitamins, potassium, calcium, and numerous phytochemical fighters for heart, lung, and intestinal health. As if that weren't recommendation enough, broccoli rabe requires less cooking than broccoli. My favorite rabe preparation is to cut it into pieces, rinse, and add to hot olive oil in which several cloves of garlic have been browned. Stir the vegetable in the oil, add a small bit of water, cover, then steam for several minutes—a marvelous side dish.

Turnips

The turnip is really two vegetables, a root crucifer and a leafy green. Both leaves and roots were used as food before the dawn of agriculture. Cultivation dates back some four thousand years, to the cradle of civilization in the Middle East. Turnips remained an important food crop for centuries, grown for both human food and animal fodder. One reason for their importance, apart from nutrition, was that they keep well in outdoor storage over the winter even in cold climates. Farmers could therefore keep their animals well fed over the winter, and could feed themselves as well. As a food for humans, however, turnips eventually lost popularity to the potato, which was embraced especially in northern Europe during the eighteenth century.

PowerFoods

But the turnip is back, thanks to a renewed interest in the health benefits of vegetables, and thanks, too, to its versatility. The turnip is a powerhouse of protein, with a cup of turnip greens equal in protein content to that of a cup of cooked cereal, at one-fourth the calories. It's also rich in vitamins, especially Vitamins C and E and the B vitamin known as folic acid, in minerals like calcium and iron, and in the cancer-fighting antioxidants.

As a recipe ingredient, turnip's delicate flavor means it combines well with just about anything. Peel, dice, or slice the roots and simmer for 12 to 15 minutes. Or mash turnips with boiled potatoes and season with a little curry powder, or with onions, or with scallions, or with the spice of your choice. Turnip root flavors soups, stews, and casseroles.

Rutabagas

The rutabaga is sometimes called the "superturnip," but in fact it is larger, rounder, and another species altogether. A Scandinavian favorite, rutabagas are root-only vegetables; the leaves are inedible. Its flavor is more pronounced than that of turnip. Ounce for ounce, it is more nutritious than turnip, but it can be served in the same way as turnips—mashed and combined with potatoes or carrots, or added to soups, stews, and casseroles. Rutabagas require twice the cooking time of turnips and they are well worth it.

Picking a Bunch of Greens

Mustard greens grow wild throughout the world, peaking in late winter and early spring, and while their seeds are used as a spice or ground and mixed with water and wine, the greens are delicious raw, steamed, boiled, or sautéed, especially with garlic. An excellent source of calcium and iron in addition to the phytochemicals, mustard greens are medicinal for the lungs and colon.

Leafy chicory comes in red as well as green and is esteemed as a medicinal herb for liver irregularities, as a blood purifier, and to nourish the heart and circulatory system. Chicory is also an excellent source of potassium, calcium, and Vitamin A. A popular salad vegetable, chicory can be blanched to reduce the bitter flavor.

Ogden Nash once opined that "Parsley's gharsley," but this relative of rosemary and cilantro has long been believed to contain magical properties. The Greeks thought it stimulated the brain; in the Middle Ages, parsley seed poultices were used to banish freckles; and Beatrix Potter's Peter Rabbit ate parsley to cure his upset stomach.

Peter Rabbit was right: Parsley is good for you. It's full of iron, and its phytochemical content includes coumarins, flavonoids, terpenes, and the carotenoids. Parsley is a good diuretic, is helpful against the symptoms of premenstrual syndrome, and works as an antiaging agent. Its uses as a garnish and in salads and soups are well known; try parsley in yogurt as a dip, as the base for pesto, or in salsa. Or do as the Italians do: Discard the stems and sauté whole handfuls of parsley in olive oil and minced garlic, and eat as a vegetable.

Dandelion greens are coming into their own these days; in fact, they're becoming downright trendy. And no wonder: They combine topflight health benefits with topflight taste. The Center for Science in the Public Interest ranks this humble weed high on its list of healthiest vegetables. Dandelion greens not only boast more calcium than whole milk, they're also loaded with antioxidants. The Chinese have long looked to dandelion poultices to treat breast cancers, and like chicory, these greens cleanse liver and blood. Their pungent taste, meanwhile, adds zing to any salad, and they are delicious sautéed with onions, garlic, and a touch of sage. They are best and most abundant in early spring. Collect the wild greens before the plant blossoms from an area that has not been sprayed with insecticide or weed-killer. For milder, less bitter greens, pick from a shady area or from an area partially mulched with leaves. Alternatively, pick up some dandelion greens at your local produce stand or specialty vegetable market. The commercially cultivated variety are lighter in color and with a thicker leaf than the weed on your front lawn.

Another new fad among greens—perhaps truly deserving of the term *designer greens*—is mesclun, which is increasingly available in supermarkets from sea to shining sea. It is a melange made up predominantly of the leaves of various baby lettuces, some bitter and some sweet; the mix can range from oak leaf and lamb's tongue lettuces to nasturtium petals. Because the leaves are picked when the greens are very young, they are particularly tender, and particularly tasty. Mesclun is found in the produce section of the market; although it does come prepackaged, it is more common to find it in a bin from which you scoop up your portion with tongs. Mesclun makes a superb salad, adding its very definite tastes, both the sweet and the tart.

All these greens, not to mention the likes of bok choy and Chinese cabbage that are becoming so popular here in the United States, are easy and highly rewarding gardening candidates, even for the ungreenest thumb imaginable. They like cool weather, can be planted as soon as the ground is ready, germinate quickly, require only sun and water, and shoot up within ten days, ready to eat. At a time of year when our bodies are in particular need of the kind of replenishment these PowerFoods offer, they can be as close as the backyard or the flowerpot on the window sill.

Chapter 7

Mushrooms

In recent years, edible mushrooms have been shown to have antitumor and cholesterol-lowering properties. The phytochemical lentinan found in mushrooms is especially protective.

—DR. B. HUANG
DEPARTMENT OF BIOLOGY
HONG KONG CHINESE UNIVERSITY

*t*he mushroom is neither vegetable nor fruit. It lacks the bright colors of other PowerFoods, foods that by their very appearance offer an image of robust good health. This PowerFood is a fungus, a mold that grows in the dark, that has neither roots nor leaves, that yields neither flower nor seed, that subsists on organic matter—often dead organic matter. In the eyes of many people, there's nothing pretty about mushrooms, and the fact that many wild varieties are highly toxic, even fatal, only exacerbates their fearsome image.

To others, of course, mushrooms are very beautiful indeed. They are the height of culinary distinction, an ingredient used lavishly and to perfection in what are perhaps the "hautest" of the world's hautes cuisines—the French, Italian, and Chinese.

Long a staple of the Chinese stir-fry, a traditional accompaniment to pasta of all shapes, and, in France, a stand-alone dish that is its own reward, the mushroom has been considered a delicacy at least since the time of the Egyptian pharoahs, who declared the wild mushroom a royal food. The French made the champignon their own in the seventeenth century, when they began to cultivate mushrooms in caves. Over the next two centuries, commercial mushroom cultivation grew and spread throughout Europe, then crossed the Atlantic to the United States, where farmers in Pennsylvania and Delaware made their states centers of American mushroom production. Today, most commercially cultivated mushrooms are grown in controlled environments in specially designed buildings. From being a costly delicacy fit for kings and obtainable by very few others, they have become an affordable food available year-round in fresh or dried form.

The Power of This PowerFood

The growing use and popularity of the mushroom in the United States is due partly to an ever more sophisticated American palate, partly to the simple fact that more varieties of edible mushroom have made their way into American markets, and partly to the increasingly dramatic news of their nutritive value.

Mushrooms have no chlorophyll, Vitamin C, or carotenoids, but they make up for this omission by being filled with B vitamins, copper, and other minerals. They are a source of protein and fiber, and they are low in calories, a fact that surprises many people. Yet it is their medicinal properties, long made use of in traditional Chinese medical practice, that have recently been the subject of scientific research and analysis.

I am not speaking here of the pharmacological activity of so-called "magic" mushrooms, the perception-altering delirium claimed by those who like having their perceptions altered. Despite the ritual use of mushrooms in certain religious ceremonies of Native American tribes, and despite such literary associations as that presumed for Lewis Carroll and *Alice's Adventures in Wonderland,* this kind of pharmacological activity has a toxic origin and toxic result. There's nothing healthful about it.

What laboratory researchers and clinical trials have been confirming is that certain mushrooms act as immunomodulators—that is, they enhance the function and activity of the immune system. In addition, mushrooms can serve as a powerful anticoagulant, preventing abnormal blood clotting and thus helping to stave off coronary problems. These powers are probably why traditional Chinese medicine has long prescribed this PowerFood as a tonic, to suppress tumors, to inactivate viruses, and to enhance longevity.

What appears to be one of the key sources of this power is a phytochemical called lentinan, a booster of the immune system that exhibits strong antitumor activity and enhances resistance to bacterial, viral, and parasite infections.

A Mushroom Sampler

There are an estimated 38,000 varieties of mushrooms, many of them highly toxic and even fatal. The toxic varieties can damage the heart, liver, and kidneys and can cause anaphylactic shock. The conclusion is obvious: Leave wild mushroom picking to expert mycologists; gather your PowerFood power from your local market.

The variety of edible mushrooms left after you subtract the poisonous ones is still staggering. In France, where mushrooms are an adored and treasured food, I was once lucky enough to eat a single dish containing fourteen separate varieties of mushroom. One mark of the growing popularity of mushrooms in the United States is that, where it was once possible to find button mushrooms or nothing, you can today shop for upwards of a dozen different varieties. Because these varieties proffer a range of tastes and textures, and because mushrooms have an affinity to such a wide range of foods, it means no end of possibilities for taking in the phytochemical power this PowerFood offers.

In fact, the most widely available mushroom, the white or brown button mushroom also known as agaricus, is perhaps the least effectual, phytochemically speaking. You can realize greater disease-fighting benefits and more pronounced taste if you substitute shiitake, oyster, or portobello mushrooms for the agaricus. In fact, all of these are interchangeable in recipes, allowing for experimentation among mushroom tastes and textures.

The shiitake mushroom, also called the oak, Chinese, or Black Forest mushroom, was once strictly an import. Today, shiitakes are grown in numerous parts of the United States, cultivated on artificial logs. They range in color from tan to dark brown and have broad caps. Although shiitakes have a meaty texture, their flavor is rather delicate and somewhat woodsy. They are great in stir-fries and go well in pastas and soups.

The shiitake is one of the most therapeutic of the mushrooms. Laboratory research shows that the pharmacological activity of the shiitake stimulates the immune system. In clinical trials, it has been shown to be a powerful antiviral, to lower blood cholesterol, improve circulation, even block some of the bad effects of saturated fats.

The oyster mushroom, so named for its fluted shell shape and soft brown or gray color, is an excellent accompaniment for seafood. It is best eaten cooked rather than raw.

The maitake mushroom is just now beginning to be known in the United States. Maitake tinctures, teas, and extracts are available in health food and natural food shops, and dried maitake (and sometimes the fresh) can be found in oriental markets. The maitake is indigenous to northern Japan, where it has long been a staple of traditional herbal medicine. Its name means "dancing mushroom"—a reference to the joyful reaction of people who found it in the woods. During Japan's feudal era, maitakes could be exchanged for their weight in silver, and they remain today a valuable and costly mushroom.

Their true value, as demonstrated in recent laboratory research in Japan, is that "of all mushrooms studied, maitake has the strongest activity in tumor growth inhibition,"* as one study put it. The source of the maitake's value, the research shows, is the phytochemical called D-fraction, which enhances the immune system and acts to suppress tumors. Maitake also works as an antihypertensive, antidiabetes, antiobesity, and antihepatitis agent, and it is currently under study for its anti–HIV properties. But it is as a cancer inhibitor that D-fraction—and the maitake mushroom containing it—are best known and most useful.

The portobello mushroom is the classic humungous fungus—a larger relative of the agaricus. It is very flavorful; in fact, it is known for tasting like a rich steak when grilled. Nutritionist Kathie Swift tells of "converting" a meat lover whose diet was, in Kathie's words, "a nutritional trainwreck, especially considering his history of heart disease, high cholesterol, gout, and arthritis." She taught him to grill mar-

*Nanba, Hiroaki. "Maitake D-fraction Healing and Preventing Potentials for Cancer." Townsend Letter for Doctors & Patients. February/March 1996.

inated portobello mushrooms, and he was so satisfied by their taste and texture that he willingly tried other mushrooms—and other PowerFoods.

The enoki is a creamy white mushroom with fragile, spaghettilike stems and tiny caps. It is generally eaten raw or as a garnish for salads, soups, and sandwiches. Originally, enoki mushrooms were found only in Japan, where they grew wild on dead trees; today, they are cultivated in this country. Like the shiitakes, enoki mushrooms have been shown to stimulate the immune system of animals; moreover, in a region of Japan where they are commercially grown and widely eaten, the rate of cancer is particularly low.

The wood ear is also known as the black tree fungus or, by the Chinese, the tree ear, *mo-er.* These mushrooms have particularly potent anticoagulant properties; they keep blood platelets from sticking together. For that reason, they have been an important prescription in traditional Eastern medicines, used like aspirin to thin the blood and considered also to retard the growth of cancerous tumors.

Buying, Storing, Handling, and Preparing Mushrooms

In the market, look for firm, meaty mushrooms, and sniff them for a pleasant, "earthy" fragrance.

Once you get them home, store mushrooms, unwashed and unpeeled, in a cool place. The mushroom storage dilemma is that dry mushrooms shrivel, while soggy ones decay. The best bet for balance is to store mushrooms on a refrigerator shelf—not in the crisper, which can be humid, or in any closed bin where they will not get the benefits of air circulation. Cover them gently with a damp paper towel or cheesecloth to retain what moisture they do have.

Shelf life will vary. Agaricus, shiitake, and portobello mushrooms will last about a week. Enokis can last from three to four days, oyster mushrooms two to three days. It's a good idea, therefore, to buy only as much as you actually need, and to rotate your supply so that the first purchased are the first eaten. If the mushrooms begin to darken, or if their caps start to open, they can be sautéed and frozen for future use in soups, stews, or casseroles, where their appearance will be secondary to their taste.

To prepare mushrooms, wipe them gently with a soft brush or cloth and trim the stems. That's really all that's needed. If you have sliced up raw mushrooms in advance of serving them, dip the slices in lemon juice to preserve their color.

Cooking and Serving Mushrooms

Mushrooms are good just about any way you cook them. Be guided by the fact that they are very absorbent and soak up whatever liquid they are in, so, among other things, don't soak them before cooking. In Sweden, according to my Swedish husband, the word for mushroom ("svamp") is also the word for sponge. The longer mushrooms cook, the more water they lose and the chewier they will be; shorter cooking time yields a more delicate texture. Mushrooms should not be cooked in aluminum pans, which they will discolor; use steel, ceramic, or enamel.

In sautéing mushrooms, as a rule of thumb, figure one tablespoon of oil for each eight ounces of mushrooms. Here's a suggestion: Add a sprinkle of herbs like rosemary or tarragon to the oil for heightened flavor. Mushrooms can also be steamed, baked, or roasted without any added fat. To roast, place them in a shallow baking pan and roast at 375° F. for about 15 minutes, stirring occasionally (You might want to spray your baking pan with a nonstick vegetable spray.) Of course, mushrooms are great broiled in the oven or grilled on the barbecue. Thread them on skewers with a range of summer PowerFoods— squash, peppers, garlic—then grill. As a stir-fry ingredient, mushrooms require only three to four minutes of cooking. They can even be microwaved; two to three minutes at 100 percent will do it.

Cooked mushrooms take seasonings especially well. Try tarragon, basil, lemon juice, and pepper. Mushrooms with garlic and onions are a classic Mediterranean dish, as well as a PowerFood special, that can also flavor pasta sauces, stir-fries, and poultry dishes. Try adding some dill and plain yogurt to cooked mushrooms. Fill mushroom caps with puréed versions of such PowerFoods as peas or spinach. Add broiled mushrooms to rice, barley, or other grains. Sautéed in a little olive oil, mushrooms are a superb pasta enhancement.

Dried mushrooms retain the punch of fresh mushrooms, but they must be reconstituted before being served. Since the drying has intensified their flavor concentration, dried mushrooms are better as a seasoning than as a stand-alone dish. Your best bet, for both versatility of eating and disease-fighting power, is the range of fresh mushrooms in the market in any season.

Chapter 8

Sea Vegetables

Modern science confirms that seaweed is one of nature's all-around pharmaceutical miracles, full of chemicals that can accomplish everything from warding off and treating several types of cancer, lowering blood cholesterol and blood pressure, thinning the blood, preventing ulcers, killing bacteria, and even curing constipation.

—JEAN CARPER
AUTHOR OF *THE FOOD PHARMACY*

*O*kay, this is the funny one. All the other PowerFoods in this book are foods you've most likely eaten all your life. There is nothing unfamiliar about fruits and vegetables, bread and beans, nuts and seeds. The only thing new is to put these foods first, creating a way of eating that emphasizes PowerFoods. Seaweed, on the other hand, is an exotic stranger to most American diets.

You may have encountered sea vegetables in sushi, which uses a black red algae called nori to wrap the sushi. Agar-agar, also called kanten, is a common thickener for desserts, puddings, and pie fillings. If you've ever traveled in Ireland or Scotland, Denmark or Iceland, chances are you have eaten foods flavored with dulse, a kind of sea moss, or have nibbled on the flatbreads, often called laverbread, made of the nori algae.

Sea vegetables are typically used in emulsifiers—you may have eaten some in ice cream. They are used in the fodder fed to farm animals, in paints and paper, in such beauty aids as creams and lotions, and in many other products that are familiar household items. So you have certainly been around sea vegetables, even if they have not been a staple of your diet.

Not surprisingly, sea vegetables *are* staple foods of societies living near the sea, and they have been so for many thousands of years. Plant life began in the oceans, and the undersea strand where water meets land still constitutes a rich source of these PowerFoods. There is evidence of sea vegetables in Paleolithic burial sites. Ancient Chinese medical texts prescribe sea vegetables. Medieval Japanese court poetry speaks of them. In ancient Hawaii, they were the food of the nobility. In Iceland, laws codifying the harvesting rights to wild dulse date back a thousand years. Today, sea vegetables remain an important food source and are prized for their healing properties among peoples of the northern Atlantic and throughout the islands of the Pacific as well.

The Power of This PowerFood

Sea vegetables are exceptionally concentrated packages of nutrients and phytochemicals. They contain vitamins, are high in fiber, and have small amounts of protein. Mostly, sea vegetables are a rich source of such minerals as potassium, calcium, magnesium, iron, and iodine. Kathie Swift says that even a few flakes sprinkled into a bean chili or soup can boost your mineral intake dramatically. She cites the example of a client who was taking in only 1400 calories per day but had a vitamin and mineral content well above most other diets at that calorie level. The nutritional superstar was the sea vegetables she used daily. In fact, Kathie's analysis of the client's diet without the sea vegetables showed several nutrients in short supply.

Thanks to their phytochemical power, sea vegetables are anti-inflammatory and tumor-suppressing. Their phytochemical content also includes the carotenoids and flavonoids, the most powerful of the antioxidants.

Researchers have suggested that the ubiquitous presence of sea vegetables in the Japanese diet may be why the incidence of breast cancer in Japanese women is one-sixth that in American women. Sea vegetables have been shown in the test tube and in laboratory animals to suppress colon cancer and to boost the immune system. A drink or broth made from kombu, a brown alga, reduces hypertension and can help prevent strokes. Japanese scientists believe that substances in nori fight numerous disease-causing bacteria, combat ulcers, and serve as an anticoagulant.

Certainly folk medicine has long used "kelp," really a brown alga but used as a catchall word for sea vegetables, to treat such ailments as indigestion, arthritis, stress, skin diseases, asthma, even constipation. And ongoing research into the supranutritive power of sea vegetables seems to be confirming its healing potential.

Putting Sea Vegetables in Your Diet

Sea vegetables tend to have a salty taste. Fresh, they taste like salty greens. As dry powder or flakes, they are a salty flavoring to be sprinkled over food. In fact, that is a common and logical use for dried sea vegetables. They are convenient additions to soups and salads, go well with other vegetables, and can even be brewed.

For the most part, it's still necessary to go to a health food store, a Japanese market, or a large produce market or specialty store to find sea vegetables, although they are becoming more widely available. Dulse, nori, kombu, and agar-agar are the most commonly sold of the sea vegetables. Typically, they come in powder, granules, sheets, and flakes.

Agar-agar is less a food than a gelling agent, used to firm or thicken liquids or mixtures. Agar sets at room temperature, and it will gel such enzyme-containing liquids as pineapple juice and papaya juice—something a gelatin thickener will not do. The thinner the liquid you are gelling, the less agar you will need. Agar is calorie-free, color-free, and flavor-free, but it is full of minerals, vitamins, and phytochemicals.

Dulse, which comes as curled, dried strips, can be eaten right out of the bag. It can be chopped and added to salads, soups, stews, stir-fries, or casseroles. It is tasty sautéed with root vegetables. Bake dulse on a sheet in the middle rack of the oven for about three minutes at 300° F., then crumble it onto grains or vegetables or use in such ground meat dishes as meat loaf. The Scots make soup from dulse.

Nori typically comes in sheets or strips. Toasted, it can be used to replace toasted dulse in soups, vegetable platters, and grain dishes.

Kombu is typically used for making stocks. It is thought to aid in the digestion of legumes because it contains a natural glutamatic acid that tenderizes the legumes, enhancing their flavor while doing so. Of course, if you do not tolerate monosodium glutamate (MSG), you may have the same problem with the natural glutamatic acid in kombu.

Wakame and *arame* are two other sea vegetables available packaged in dried form. Wakame is similar to kombu and is typically cooked in stir-fries or soups, especially miso, the staple of Japanese breakfasts. Marinated wakame serves as a bed for fish or can be used in salads. Arame, curly black seaweed tendrils, makes a wonderful stuffing or salad ingredient after it has been soaked in water. Sauté arame to close the edges and retain the flavor, add carrots, onions, soy sauce, and a dash of water for a wonderful side dish.

It may take some boldness to add sea vegetables to your diet. Once you do, their usefulness, driven by your ingenuity, can be as wide as the ocean from which they come—and the payback in disease-fighting and antiaging power can be substantial.

Chapter 9

Garlic and Company

Several epidemiological studies show that people who eat a lot of garlic and onions have lower risk of cancers of the gastrointestinal tract, such as stomach and colon cancer.
—DR. MICHAEL WARGOVICH,
M.J. ANDERSON CANCER CENTER, HOUSTON, TX

The sulfur compounds in garlic may be linked to lower cancer incidence and improved immune status. Garlic should also be used for its flavor as part of a low-fat diet.
—AMERICAN INSTITUTE FOR CANCER RESEARCH

Garlic may also protect against heart disease and stroke by interfering with the formation of blood clots and by reducing cholesterol.
—MEGHAN FLYNN, M.S., R.D.

*t*he Chinese refer to the alliums—garlic, onions, leeks, shallots, scallions, and chives—as "jewels among vegetables," and prize them for their health-giving properties and for their sharp taste and smell. In fact, just as the intense *colors* of fruits and vegetables give evidence of heightened phytochemical power, the stronger the *smell* of garlic and its relatives, the more effective their healing powers.

Garlic and company, as I like to think of the allium family, are the quintessential folk remedies of history and legend. Evidence of garlic as both food and health potion goes back at least as far as the Sumerian civilization of the fourth millennium B.C. Garlic accompanied Egypt's

89

King Tutankhamen to his tomb back around 1400 B.C., and thanks to the dry sands of Egypt, it was preserved there virtually intact, to be found when the tomb was opened in 1922.

Egyptian physicians, who were justifiably renowned throughout the ancient world, recommended the onion for eight thousand separate ailments and prescribed garlic as a remedy for complaints ranging from headache to physical weakness. It was to guard against weakness, in fact, that Egyptian overseers fed garlic to the Hebrew slaves laboring on the great pyramids, and when these same Hebrews were freed from Egypt to wander in the desert, it was leeks and onions and garlic they pined for.

Hippocrates, the ancient Greek physician known as the father of Western medicine, recommended garlic as a laxative and diuretic, and he prescribed it as a cure for tumors of the uterus. In Shakespearean England, it was regarded as an aphrodisiac. In ancient Rome, the elder Pliny listed sixty-one illnesses for which garlic was a remedy, including gastrointestinal disorders, snakebite, asthma, ulcers, loss of appetite, hemorrhoids, consumption, and tumors.

Roman soldiers on long marches were given garlic to keep up their strength. Many centuries later, in 1864, General Ulysses S. Grant told the War Department in Washington: "I will not move my army without onions!" He believed them particularly effective against the diseases of hot climates, like that of the American South, where he expected to move his troops in force. In World Wars I and II, garlic was used against typhus and dysentery and as a battlefield dressing to keep wounds from becoming septic.

Leeks, large-scale scallionlike plants that combine the smells of both garlic and onions but are sweeter than either, are the national symbol of Wales. Marco Polo brought the chive west from China along with the noodle; Chinese and Japanese physicians for centuries had used chives as well as garlic as a treatment for high blood pressure. Ancient medical tracts of India ascribe to garlic and onions preventive properties against heart disease and rheumatism.

Normans and Saxons both wore garlic close to the skin to ward off colds (and black magic) and they ate it as a seasoning on their food to ward off catarrh and worms and to "cleanse the blood." Peasant farmers across Europe from ancient times to modern believed that just about any of the allium plants could deter aphids and mildew. An old Ukrainian deterrent to the debilities of old age calls for a nightly sip of a drink combining a pound of garlic with the juice of twenty-four lemons, covered and left to stand for twenty-four days. In the Basque culture, a cough remedy handed down from long ago calls for pouring dark honey over sliced Spanish onions, straining the mixture, then mixing the onion and honey syrup with water and lemon juice. Traditional medicine in the Far East typically used onions and garlic to treat tuberculosis.

And of course, most of the world's cooking uses all these plants as a basic and important culinary flavoring. Flavor, of course, is a matter of taste, but science is a matter of demonstrated evidence, and science today is confirming that most of what history has attributed to the alliums is true: Garlic, onions, leeks, shallots, scallions, and chives have powerful antiaging and antidisease properties.

What They Are, Where They're From

All the garlic and company PowerFoods are bulb plants; this simply means that their buds are underground. Garlic's bulb is wrapped in an outer skin; the bulb comprises several sections, called cloves, each of which has its own papery covering. Garlic comes in numerous varieties and is available year-round. It is often imported from Latin America; domestically, California is the biggest producer.

Garlic is a staple of the kitchens of the Mediterranean, the Middle East, India, and China. Americans consume about 250 million pounds of garlic a year, and its use is increasing. Attendance is up at the classic Garlic Festival in Gilroy, California, heart of garlic production in the United States, and garlic festivals are proliferating from Arizona to Virginia. In Saugerties, New York, a festival that boasted 125 attendants the first year it was held in 1989 attracted 45,000 people five years later.

Leeks are also gaining ground in the United States, although they are still not as well known a food here as in Europe, particularly in France, Belgium, and the Netherlands, the world's leading leeks producers. Here in the States, leeks are grown in California, Florida, and New Jersey, and they are available all year.

Onions come in so many varieties that at any given season, some section of the country is growing or harvesting some form of onion. Spring and summer onions are grown from fall to spring in the warm-weather states, while storage onions are harvested in late summer and early fall in the northern zones. The result is that onions are available throughout the year in ample quantities and in great variety.

Shallots, smaller than onions and more gentle than garlic, resemble both. They are grown commercially in New Jersey and New York, and they are also available, at higher cost, from France, where they are beloved. Their flavor is milder and more delicate than that of the other alliums.

With their hollow green shoots, chives look like a grassier scallion, which is pretty much what they are. As a food, chives are treasured for these green shoots, rather than for their bulbs, which are minuscule. Chives are grown commercially in some thirty states, as well as in many backyard gardens.

The Power of This PowerFood

All the garlic and company PowerFoods are high-voltage bulbs, downright incandescent in their power to prevent disease and resist the effects of aging. Start with the studies, clinical trials, and experiments proceeding apace around the world:

A study of elderly women in Iowa found that those who ate garlic more than once a week had half the incidence of colon cancer that afflicted women who never ate it. Studies in China and Italy find that those who eat both garlic and onions exhibit half the incidence of stomach cancer. In Houston, Texas, experiments with onion oils have yielded cancer-inhibiting results. Prostate cancer cells have been shown to grow more slowly when exposed to the dominant garlic phytochemical, allicin; similar inhibiting properties have been shown on cancers of the breast, liver, and colon.

In experiments in Munich, onion extract given to sufferers of bronchial asthma has succeeded in inhibiting the disease; applied directly to the skin, it has helped allergic patients ward off their usual reactions to various substances.

In Britain and Germany, clinical trials have demonstrated that large doses of garlic can be as effective as drugs in lowering cholesterol. Experiments in Kansas have shown that in addition to lowering cholesterol, garlic cripples cholesterol's ability to clog arteries; it also helps lower blood pressure. Other research has shown that it can dissolve blood clots. Cardiology researchers at Tagore Medical College in India have found that garlic can even help dissolve blockages in arteries, thus both prolonging life and preventing subsequent heart attacks.

In Japan, garlic and company have been shown to restore brain functioning and immune functioning in elderly rats; further research continues to test the ancient folkloric tradition that this PowerFood resists senility. In Florida, investigators have found evidence that garlic extract bolsters the immune system's ability to ward off infections. In France, researchers at the Pasteur Institute regard the alliums as having antidepressant, antianxiety, antistress properties. And so on, and on, and on: Impressive evidence continues to mount. Meanwhile, other investigators are exploring what it is about garlic and company that produces such results.

To be sure, this is a PowerFood rich in Vitamins A, B, and C and containing such minerals as calcium, potassium, and iron. Scientists are discovering that garlic and company are exceptionally abundant in phytochemicals, particularly in the blood-cleansing, cholesterol-lowering saponins; in such flavonoid antioxidants as quercetin; and above all, in the organosulfurs, especially the pungent allicin, from which the allium genus takes its name.

So numerous are the chemicals in garlic and company, so intense their concentration, that these plants constitute nothing less than what scientists call an adaptogenic class—that is, they spawn mechanisms that always seek equilibrium in response to all environmental changes, and that therefore are always blocking attempts to compromise the immune system. In other words, the chemicals in this PowerFood suppress deterioration by detoxifying potentially toxic attacks and by preventing diseases of all kinds. These are the kind of fighter PowerFoods you want on your side.

Their fighting power starts when garlic and company release allicin—and a pungent smell—once the skin of the bulb is cut. The very act of cutting or slicing stimulates enzymatic action on the organosulfur amino acids. This action yields a number of volatile compounds. Anyone who has ever chopped an onion knows one side of this volatility: the irritation to skin, eyes, and tongue, a milder version of the grave toxic irritation sulfuric acid can cause. Cooking weakens this reaction, making both the smell and taste of the allium considerably milder, while still, of course, adding taste to whatever is cooking. It's that smelly, irritating enzymatic action, however, that is the healing power of this PowerFood, and the power is considerable.

Another potent compound unleashed by the process is diallyl disulfide, organosulfur that acts as a blocking and suppressing agent and stimulates production of a detoxification enzyme called glutathione-S-transferase.

What diallyl disulfide blocks and suppresses and what glutathione-S-transferase detoxifies is a range of ailments and syndromes. The net effect is an infection-fighting, heart-happy, lung-protecting, cancer-preventing, blood-cleansing PowerFood. Out of the laboratory and in your diet, this PowerFood works as a blood-thinning anticoagulant, as a decongestant and expectorant, as a lowerer of bad cholesterol, raiser of good cholesterol, cancer-suppressing antioxidant, and as a broad-spectrum antibiotic that literally destroys bacteria, fungus, parasites, and viruses.

In other words, garlic, onions, leeks, shallots, scallions, and chives do just what the ancients said they did. It's just that today, science and technology let us know why we should go back to the future, phytochemically speaking.

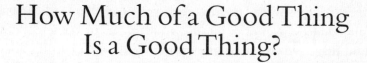

How Much of a Good Thing
Is a Good Thing?

Laboratory studies and clinical trials again and again show the effectiveness of this PowerFood when taken in large amounts—probably larger amounts than many people find tasty or comfortable. Too much, however (especially too much garlic) can make the mouth burn, distress the stomach, even cause diarrhea and bloating. Raw garlic in high doses can be toxic, although there are no ill effects from cooked garlic.

As to garlic supplements, trying to gain the benefits of any PowerFood through supplements is a bad idea as has been emphasized throughout this book. Although garlic supplements do retain the active ingredients of the real food, you can easily overdose on them. Moreover, even taking something as benign as aspirin could, in combination with the garlic supplement, inhibit blood clotting to a dangerous degree. The best way to take what PowerFoods have to offer you is by making them part of a varied diet. In the case of garlic and company, you may want to increase your intake to augment the proportion of this PowerFood to others in your diet. But do so in real food form, not in pills.

Buying, Storing, and Serving
Garlic and Company

Buy garlic and shallots from loose bins where you can examine them. In both cases look for a solid, plump bulb with unbroken outside skin. If the skin flakes off, or if the bulb feels too light in the hand, it may be desiccated inside. Garlic, onions, and shallots should be firm and free of sprouts.

Store the bulbs in a cool place and in a dark jar to avoid sprouting, which draws off some of the pungency from the bulb, thus diminishing its phytochemical punch. Both garlic and shallots should last at least a month.

The individual cloves of the garlic bulb break apart easily once you peel off the outer layers of skin; just snap them off the base. To peel individual cloves of garlic, use your fingers or the tried-and-true method practiced by chefs: line up the cloves on a cutting board, set the flat of a knife across them, then press down on the knife with your fist, splitting the peels. Alternatively, one of the newer kitchen gadgets is a piece of tubing sold as a garlic peeler; it works wonderfully. Treat shallots as you do onions.

Raw garlic is garlic at its most potent, both in terms of taste and smell and in terms of healing properties. Sautéing garlic cuts back on this potency somewhat, and boiling or baking turns it almost sweet. Baked or roasted garlic has a nutty flavor and buttery consistency and makes a good spread for bread or crackers.

Garlic is central to so many of the world's cuisines, with uses so numerous and so varied, that about the only place it does not belong is in sweet desserts—at least, not so far as I know. It is great in salads, makes a superb flavoring for bread, jazzes up meat and poultry dishes, is delicious in soup, and adds both taste and disease-fighting power to just about every recipe you can devise.

When shopping for leeks, look for moist, crisp, unblemished bunches. Limp, dried-out leaves are a sign that the leeks have been stored for too long. The same goes for leeks you store at home; when the leaves are dry, the leeks are past their prime. Unlike scallion bulbs, the bulbs of leeks should not be "bulbous;" rather, they should be straight and narrow. If the bulbs are too thick, the leeks may be woody. Store leeks in the refrigerator, as they are perishable. To prepare them, trim the leeks top and bottom, removing limp outer leaves and the rootlets at the base. Slice lengthwise before rinsing thoroughly under cold running water to remove all grit. If serving whole, pay extra attention to rinsing between the leaf layers.

Leeks can be steamed or boiled and served whole for a side dish or appetizer. And they are perhaps most famously served braised, flavored with lemon juice, or combined with other vegetables. Leeks also take well to soups and stews, and they are a good substitute for onions in just about any recipe. I love them in soups, but also in salad: sliced raw leeks look beautiful and have a gentle zing.

Onions, from the most bitingly pungent to the sweetest Vidalias, are typically sold loose or in mesh bags. They should smell mild; the pungency is only in the taste, so if the onions you're buying smell strong, they are probably in a state of early decay; put them back. The onions should feel dry and solid; avoid any specimens with soft spots, sprouts, or dark patches, which may be a sign of mold.

As with garlic, onions are best stored in a cool, dark, well-ventilated place. Storage onions, those harvested in late summer, should last three to four weeks; the spring and summer onions last only about two weeks. Onions will also store well in the crisper of the refrigerator.

There is no end to the ways onions may be prepared and served, from baking to boiling to braising to sautéing to blanching to roasting and even microwaving, not to mention as an essential ingredient in sauces and relishes. My favorite is boiled onions, simple as that is, but when I'm in the mood for a sweet treat, I will pop them into a 350°F. oven and roast them for 45 minutes to an hour. Roasting any root vegetable or bulb brings out its inherent sweetness.

In summer, I enjoy a salad of sliced red or Spanish onions alternating with slices of fresh tomatoes, seasoned with a little olive oil, wine vinegar, and ground pepper, sprinkled with chopped fresh garlic and snippets of chives, and perhaps garnished with capers. A PowerFoods powerhouse, packed with healing effects and full of robust, seasonal taste.

How to Avoid Garlic Breath and Onion Tears

The traditional antidote to garlic breath is to eat a sprig of parsley. The French, not surprisingly, use red wine instead. Cloves, coffee, yogurt, or a glass of milk are other folkloric prescriptions. One tried and true solution to the problem is just to make sure that everyone around you is also eating garlic.

To remove the smell of garlic from your fingers, some people advise rubbing them with toothpaste. Others advise lemon and salt. You can even buy metal blocks that are meant to rub off the garlic smell; I know someone who swears by this method. Of course, when all else fails, try soap and water.

To keep from crying when you slice onions, try chilling the onions first, or hold them under cold water as you peel them. The method I prefer is to hold a piece of bread in your mouth without chewing or swallowing it. The pungent fumes, which seek moisture, hit the bread before they hit your eyes.

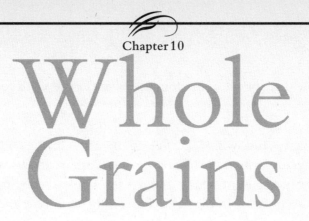

Chapter 10

Whole Grains

Consumption of whole grains reduces the risk of chronic diseases including cancer and cardiovascular disease. Components in whole grains are protective and diverse and include dietary fiber, antioxidants, phenolic compounds and the phytoestrogens with potential hormonal effects. Clearly the range of protective substances in whole grains is impressive, and the advice to consume additional whole grains is justifiable.

—DR. JOANNE SLAVIN
DEPARTMENT OF FOOD SCIENCE AND NUTRITION
UNIVERSITY OF MINNESOTA, ST. PAUL

*g*rains were the first cultivated food, the enablers of settlement and civilization, and they remain today the main food of both humans and domestic animals. They include wheat, rice, and corn—which together comprise half the world's total cropland—as well as such grasses and herbs as barley, millet, oats, buckwheat, rye, amaranth, and quinoa. The grains of these plants are their one-seeded fruits; that is, fruit and seed are united in a single kernel.

From these grains come bread, cereals, rice, and pasta—the staff of life, the rock-bottom staples of just about every cuisine on earth. Rice and noodles are the basic diet of Asians. The Italians have turned the many shapes of pasta into an art form and eat a dish of it at most meals. And just about every culture on earth boasts some form of unleavened bread that harks back to the most ancient of ancestors. Chapatis, tortillas, empanadas, and the flatbreads of the Americas all remain, quite literally, the daily bread of millions. No wonder the word for bread in many languages is the same as the word for food.

But bread and pasta, along with cereal, pretzels, rice cakes, oatmeal cookies, bran, and wheat germ—to name a few examples—are processed grain *products,* not whole grains. Corn, rice, oats, and wheat berries are examples of whole grains—the single-seeded fruit of the plants we see growing in the fields. Processing diminishes the nutritive value of whole grains. In fact, milling and refining reduce whole grains to something else altogether.

To understand this, it's useful to examine the three basic parts of a grain: endosperm, bran, and germ. The bulk of a grain (or kernel or berry)—84 percent of it—is the endosperm. Here are most of the protein and carbohydrates and most of the weight. White flour is made from the endosperm. The bran is the outer covering of the kernel, and although it's only about 14 percent of the kernel weight, it carries a disproportionate share of the nutrients, particularly the B vitamins, and most of the fiber. The smallest part of the kernel, only about 2 percent of its weight, is the germ, the embryo of the seed; it too is rich in vitamins and nutrients and contains essential fatty acids. The three parts of the kernel are separated during the milling or refining process, and the bran and germ are often removed and sold separately.

So while all grain products offer nutrients, the whole grains offer the most nutrients in the most effectively concentrated form. In following the USDA's Food Guide Pyramid, which recommends six to eleven servings of grains a day, the best recommendation is to take most of that amount in whole grains—corn, rice, oats, and the berries of the plants described in this chapter—and to go easy on the processed grain products, bread and pasta.

A note about pasta: Be aware that most commercial pasta is white bread in another form; it is processed from white flour, is not a whole grain, and is best as a bed for other PowerFoods, especially for mushrooms, tomatoes, onions, garlic, and peppers.

PowerFoods

Whole Grains and Their PowerFoods: Wheat, Corn, Rice, and Oats

Wheat is a cereal plant of the grass family. Anthropologists suspect that early humans chewed the kernel of wild wheat as a first food. They eventually learned to pound it into flour and mix it with water to make porridge. Then at a certain point, primitive man discovered that this plant could be stored and eaten over the winter and its leftovers planted in the spring to produce more. This was a breakthrough moment in history. It meant our ancestors no longer needed to forage for food but could instead stay in one place; they could develop the arts of cultivation and settlement. Thus began also the processing of grains to make them easier to cook and digest—and less nutritious to eat.

Evidence of bread wheat being cultivated in the Nile Valley of Egypt dates from 5000 B.C. By 3000 B.C., the Egyptians were baking white, leavened bread using a wild yeast present in the air. Today, some 30,000 varieties of wheat are grown throughout the world; they fall into six categories. Four of the varieties are the hard wheats—hard red spring, hard red winter, hard white, and durum, which is a very hard-kerneled wheat. The two soft wheats are soft red winter and soft white. Hard wheats are typically used for bread-making; they are higher in protein and gluten, the substance that provides the elasticity in baked products. Very hard durum wheat, whether grown in Italy or on the plains of North Dakota, is used for making pasta. Soft wheats are used to make pastries, crackers, muffins, cakes, cookies, and the flatbreads.

The milling process that creates refined white flour also reduces nutritional content. The process, comprising upwards of twenty separate steps, removes the hull and parts of the bran from the kernels, then grinds the grain into powderlike flour. In making white flour, both the germ and the bran are stripped away from the wheat kernel, leaving only the endosperm. Unrefined or whole-wheat flours retain endosperm, bran, and germ, so they contain more fiber, minerals, and phytochemicals than refined white flour.

The enriching that is a last step in the process—and that is typically marked on a package of bread—is, in white flour, partly a way of compensating for the nutrient loss of the milling and refining. In addition, enrichment fortifies the flour; that is, it adds specific amounts of iron and the B vitamins. The enrichment process was instituted in the 1940s as a response to the widespread incidence of diseases of B vitamin deficiency—pellagra and beriberi—and of iron-deficiency anemia across the United States, and to the finding that one-third of the nation had nutrient-deficient diets. Throughout the decade, state by state, the supply of U.S. white bread was steadily enriched with B vitamins and iron; pellagra and beriberi were eliminated, and the incidence of anemia dropped markedly.

In addition to flour, there are wheat foods that are not flour-based. Bulgur, for example, is made by cracking and toasting the kernel of wheat after removing some of its outer coating, known as the bran. Couscous, a staple in North African countries like Morocco, is a granular substance that is made, like pasta, from durum wheat by grinding, steaming, and drying the wheat berries. Cracked wheat, similar to bulgur, results from breaking the whole kernel. Wheat germ is the embryo of the seed and the tiniest part of the wheat kernel; it is often separated when wheat is milled into flour. Many commercial cereals are made from wheat, and it is also possible to obtain plain wheat bran and plain whole wheat kernels (the berries) to make your own cereals, or for use in soups, salads, stews, and baked goods.

Rice is generally thought to be native to the warm, moist river deltas of the Ganges, Tigris, Yangtze, and Euphrates—not surprisingly, the cradles of civilization. The Chinese began to cultivate rice about four thousand years ago, and today they still produce more than 90 percent of the world's crop. Almost all of the rice harvest in China goes to feed the Chinese; it is not surprising that the Chinese word for rice also means agriculture. Rice is also cultivated on every other continent on earth except Antarctica. Estimates are that half the world's population subsists mainly on rice.

Rice was a principal crop of the original English colonies in the New World; by 1726, it was being exported from South Carolina. It was introduced into California during the nineteenth century to feed the thousands of Chinese workers who came there to work the Gold

Rush and lay track for the transcontinental railroad. Today, California, Arkansas, and the Gulf states are the country's prime rice-producers, although you can still find Carolina rice in most markets.

As with wheat, the processing of rice removes significant nutrient content. During the refining, the outer coatings, which contain most protein and minerals, are polished away, leaving only endosperm. Brown rice, by contrast, has only its husk removed during milling; the bran remains intact—a storehouse of fiber, vitamins, minerals, and phytochemicals.

Most of the world's corn is grown in the Americas. Corn or maize is a tall-stalked grass that has been cultivated in North, Central, and South America for thousands of years. The story of how the Native American, Squanto, showed the Plymouth colonists how to plant corn, using fish as fertilizer, is one of the abiding icons of American legend.

There is evidence that various native Americans of what is today Central America had cultivated corn as early as 3400 B.C. In North America, too, the natives had for centuries grown many varieties of corn, which they ate fresh or ground for meal, as is still done today throughout the Americas. In contemporary Mexico, Indian women in the roadless back country pound the corn kernels with stone mortar and pestle, then mix in water and knead a dough, slapping and stretching it against a rock, round it into balls, then flatten out circles of dough and grill them on a griddle-stone over the fire into crisp tortillas for use as a basic bread and as the highly edible envelope they will fill with all manner of foods.

In northern Italy, the corn staple is polenta. In the United States, it can be popcorn, cornmeal for bread and puddings, succotash, hominy grits, corn chowder, and, best of all, corn on the cob.

Oats, the focus of winter breakfasts, have seen a revival of interest and attention in recent years. Although oats are believed to have been cultivated for twenty centuries, originally for medicinal purposes, they have mostly been used in animal fodder; as human food, oats appeal to people in cold, wet climates like Scotland, where oatmeal is practically the national dish.

Here in the United States, less than 5 percent of the oat crop goes to humans, although that may be changing as research increasingly suggests the nutritive value of this PowerFood—and now its supranutritive value. First, there was the oat bran frenzy, when Dr. James W. Anderson of the University of Kentucky found that blood cholesterol was substantially reduced by a daily diet containing 100 grams of oat bran. For a while, Americans were starting their mornings with oat bran muffins and coffee.

Just as that fad abated, a government report concluded that regular, old-fashioned oats—the kind used in making oatmeal, cookies, cakes, and breads—had exceptional nutritional value and potential healing capabilities. This is true however you eat your oats, because neither the bran nor the germ is removed by processing. Even the fat in oats, though higher than in many other whole grains, is mostly unsaturated, while the fiber and protein content is particularly high. The government report spurred a whole new advertising campaign by oats manufacturers, and sales increased.

If wheat, rice, corn, and oats are well-known whole grains, a number of others are becoming better known in the United States. In many cases, this is due to a greater sense of adventure in the American palate—a willingness to explore farther afield, and to enjoy a more diverse diet. As it happens, these "newer" grains are particularly potent PowerFoods.

The "Other" Whole-Grain PowerFoods

Barley, cultivated as long ago as 7000 B.C. in the dry lands of southeast Asia and the highlands of Ethiopia, is a small white grain that grows best in cool, dry climates and is a staple food in many places—for example, in such Himalayan nations as Nepal and Tibet. It was the chief bread grain in Europe until some 500 years ago. In the United States, which is the third largest barley producer on earth, it is used mostly for beer production or as animal feed.

Millet is a small, fast-growing grain, round in shape and yellow-orange in color. Although in the States it is cultivated mainly for animal feed, it is the chief cereal in parts of Africa (particularly North

Africa) and Asia (particularly India). Millet is the basis for Indian *roti* and Ethiopian *injera,* two classic flatbreads.

A pocketful of *rye* would offer a particularly potent amount of protein, although in the United States, rye is more likely to be found in rye bread or rye crackers—or in rye whisky. Rye is thought to have originated as a weed that spread westward from Asia, flourishing in wet and cold regions of eastern Europe, Russia, and Scandinavia, where it was cultivated for its grain some 1500 years ago. Rye has a robust, distinctive flavor that can make a fine addition to soups, pilafs, breads, stews, and meat dishes. In health food stores and specialty markets today, you can find this PowerFood in the form of cracked rye, rye flakes, and whole rye berries.

Despite its name, *buckwheat* is not a wheat. It is not a true grain at all; rather, buckwheat is the fruit of a leafy shrub found mostly in northern temperate climates like Russia and China. Other members of the family include sorrel and rhubarb. The name is from the Dutch *bockweit,* meaning beech wheat, and it was the Dutch who brought buckwheat to the New World. But it was in eastern Europe that buckwheat found a real home; there, roasted buckwheat groats have long been used as a porridge or side dish called, in Slavic languages, *kasha.*

Quinoa (pronounced "keen-wah") is perhaps the newest grain to be embraced by North Americans. Native to the Andes, quinoa was a staple food of the Incas and has been cultivated for some 5000 years. Like buckwheat, quinoa is not a true grain, but a leafy plant that thrives in high, arid regions and in poor soil. It has a light taste but crunchy texture, and it has the highest protein of any of the grains.

Amaranth is another South American native, although it is also indigenous to Africa, and it is another nongrain that has much in common with shrubs like pigweed and tumbleweed. It was a staple of the Aztec culture—of both the diet and the religion. The Spanish conquistadors outlawed its cultivation as a way of starving the Aztecs into submission and destroying their culture. It worked, and knowledge of amaranth virtually disappeared. Somehow, however, knowledge of this grain made its way to Asia, where its cultivation was taken up by the Indians and Chinese. Today, China is the major producer of amaranth. Slowly, amaranth is being reintroduced into the Americas as both crop and food.

The Power of This PowerFood

The reason these "newer" grains are finding their way into the American diet is the same reason that all grain foods are advocated by nutritional authorities, not to mention by physicians: their nutritional benefits.

Up to now, the nutritive value of the whole grains could be summarized by three benefits: complex carbohydrates, fiber, and vitamins. It is no accident that the U.S. Department of Agriculture puts whole grains at the base of the food pyramid, recommending anywhere from six to eleven servings of breads, cereals, rice, and pasta daily for all Americans over the age of two. What I recommend, for peak nutrition, is that of your six to eleven servings, you make the *whole grains* predominate and eat less of the processed grain products.

The complex carbohydrates (not only in whole grains but in fruits and vegetables as well) are a source of time-released energy; they are calories that won't easily turn into fat unless eaten in excess. For people concerned about weight control, the advantage of a diet high in carbohydrates is that it takes more calories to metabolize and process carbohydrates, which is a good thing. Also, a diet high in carbohydrates is more filling, so that you eat less while still getting the maximum amount of vitamins (particularly the B vitamins and Vitamin E), minerals, fiber, and phytochemicals.

The fiber content of whole grains is important in reducing cholesterol, lowering the incidence of heart disease, and ensuring gastrointestinal motility. Where diets are rich in unrefined whole grains, people have far less colon cancer, diverticulosis, hemorrhoids, even constipation than we Americans do. The fiber from whole grains provides bulk and the necessary material for microbial activity and appears to help prevent colon cancer. Whole grains provide benefits for other gastrointestinal disorders, too. For thousands of years, for example, boiled rice preparations have been a treatment for infant diarrhea, while traditional Chinese medicine prescribes rice for digestive disorders.

What newer research has made clear is the supranutritive phytochemical value of whole grains. Specifically, they are rich in the phenols, lignans, coumarins, phytosterols, and protease inhibitors. The phenols inhibit the enzymes that can mutate critical genes and cause cancer. The lignans are antioxidants, and they also appear to suppress cell mutation. The coumarins, with their first-strike capability, block cancer-causing substances before they can get started. Phytosterols knock cancer-causing estrogen hormones off their path. The pharmacological activity of protease inhibitors offers numerous benefits. For one thing, they appear to lower cholesterol; populations whose diets are very rich in barley, for example, show extremely low incidence of heart disease. Protease inhibitors have also been shown to slow down cancer, and they appear to have antiviral properties.

Buying, Preparing, and Serving Whole Grains

Except, of course, for corn, most grains are sold in boxes or sacks that are (or should be) clearly marked with a freshness date. If you do buy grains from open bins, they should be dry, fresh-smelling, and free of dust, pebbles, and debris. Package them in tightly closed containers or lockable plastic bags and store them in the refrigerator where they will last up to five months; stored at room temperature, grains will last only about one month. Frozen grains will keep almost indefinitely.

Most grains can be either simmered, steamed, or baked. Some, like amaranth, can be popped. The basic preparation is simmering: Add the grain to boiling water or other liquid, allow the water to return to a simmer, and cook without stirring, as stirring can make the grains sticky. The exception is polenta, which you should not cover and which you should stir constantly. You can enhance the flavor of all these grains by roasting or toasting them lightly in a dry skillet before you cook them. This also lightens the texture of the final product. The following table presents typical cooking times for some major grains.

Kathie Swift swears by her rice cooker, not just for rice but for all types of grains, and recommends it as a good investment for the PowerFoods kitchen. Kathie also recommends enhancing the flavor of

Grains: Cooking Times and Proportions

Grains (1 cup)	Amount of Water	Cooking Time	Yield
Barley (whole)	3 cups	1 hour, 15 minutes	3½ cups
Brown rice	2 cups	45 minutes	3 cups
Buckwheat (kasha)	2 cups	15 minutes	2½ cups
Bulgur wheat	2 cups	10 to 15 minutes	2½ cups
Cracked wheat	2 cups	25 minutes	2⅓ cups
Millet	3 cups	45 minutes	3½ cups
Polenta (coarse cornmeal)	4 cups	25 minutes	3 cups
Wild rice	3 cups	1 hour or more	4 cups
Whole wheat berries	3 cups	1 hour, 30 minutes	2⅔ cups
Quinoa	2 cups	15 minutes	2½ cups

cooked grains by adding herbal tea bags to the cooking water! She says her kids are particularly fond of cranberry-orange-spice-flavored brown rice and almond sunset barley.

Oats

In the supermarket or specialty store, oats come in three or four forms: bran, groats, the steel-cut oats from Ireland or Scotland, and rolled oats. The latter, in turn, can be either whole groats (often sold as "old-fashioned"), quick-cooking, and instant. The biggest and most effective nutritional and supranutritional punch naturally comes in old-fashioned rolled oats, which cook in about five minutes; the whole groats should be picked over and rinsed before cooking. Commercially sold cold cereals like granola and muesli can be quite high in fat and calories. You can create your own by toasting rolled oats or oat flakes first, then mixing in wheat germ, bran, dried fruits, and nuts and seeds in whatever combination intrigues you.

Don't restrict your oat-eating to breakfast. Oats add texture to soup, can replace some portion of the meat in meat loaf or meatballs, are a fine addition to batters and crusts, and can be food-processed into flour for dredging poultry or fish or for use in baking.

Bulgur and Couscous

Bulgur is a fast-cooking grain with a nutty flavor and meaty texture. It makes a fine breakfast cereal and an excellent addition to salads and stuffings. Try a bulgur pilaf, a bulgur loaf, or add it to pasta sauce or chili. Couscous, which also cooks quickly, is light, fluffy, and a perfect bed for vegetables and meats. Both bulgur and couscous need only about five to ten minutes of simmering. Alternatively, just pour boiling water over the grain, cover, and let stand for 15 minutes.

Rice

Rice comes in various grain lengths, and in brown, white, aromatic, and glutinous versions. By all means, buy the brown rice, which has not had the bran removed and contains far more nutrition and supranutrition. Domestic packaged rice is reliably clean, but imported rices and those you buy in open bins should be rinsed before cooking; basmati rice should be soaked.

You needn't limit yourself to rice cooked in plain old water; it can be cooked in broth or juices, too, and with herbs, spices, and seasoning. Simmering rice in a covered pot is the conventional preparation, but it can also be cooked in an open pot or in the microwave.

Rice can be served as a main dish or side dish; with meat or vegetables; with salsa or vinaigrette; as a stuffing or a bed on which to serve something else. And as risotto or pilaf, in a soup or a pudding, in a salad or as cereal. Let your imagination be your guide.

Corn

Corn should be bought in season and, if possible, locally just after it has been picked. The husk should fit tightly and should be fresh and green. The silks should be moist and soft. If the proprietors let you, peel back the husk a bit and check to be sure that there's no rot at the end of the cob. Press a kernel or two; the skin should be taut, not tough, and the liquid should be milky.

The methods of cooking and eating corn on the cob are very often cherished family traditions, and they vary widely. Fresher is better. One friend of mine gets her water boiling and then picks the corn off the stalks in her backyard, husking as she races indoors. She tries to keep the time between picking and cooking to 30 seconds at most. She's right, because once the corn is picked, the sugar begins to turn into starch, and the corn loses some of its sweetness. Off the cob, corn kernels also combine well with other vegetables, and they are a fine addition to salads, stir-fries, and side dishes, and as the principal ingredient in a soup or chowder.

Cornmeal prepared as polenta is delicious with any number of seasonings or with such accompaniments as roasted peppers, other vegetables, or a little melted cheese. Cornmeal also makes wonderful breads, muffins, pancakes, and puddings.

Barley

Barley is more than just the other half of mushroom-and-barley soup. It makes a superb hot cereal, and it can be an ingredient in pilaf, risotto, casseroles, as a stuffing for poultry, or a filling for vegetables.

Millet

Millet is best toasted dry before cooking. It makes a good pilaf, loaf, or grainburger, and it is an excellent stuffing for vegetables or poultry.

Rye

Apart from whiskey, rye is most familiar in bread. To get the real benefit of the whole grain, however, try rye berries. Cook them like brown rice, but for about 15 minutes longer. Since rye has a strong flavor, I like to mix it with brown rice, which I add after the rye has been cooking for 15 minutes. The result is a dish with a pleasant taste and texture, considerable nutrients, and powerful phytochemical supranutrients.

Buckwheat

Buckwheat is not just a pancake flour. Its robust flavor makes it a good accompaniment to such foods as onions and mushrooms, and it is a tasty meat stuffing or vegetable filling. The most common dish, made from buckwheat groats, is kasha. Ground buckwheat flour also makes the delicious Japanese soba noodles.

Quinoa

Quinoa should be rinsed in a strainer until the water runs clear, then drained before it is cooked. It combines well with cooked vegetables, with raw vegetables in a summer salad, in a pilaf, and with such other grains as buckwheat.

Amaranth

Amaranth is best baked or steamed, or cooked along with other grains; if simmered, it tends to produce a thick porridge with a fairly sticky texture. On the other hand, that texture makes it a good thickener for soups and stews, and it is a fine stir-fry ingredient. Amaranth can also be popped. Toss and stir the grains in a skillet over high heat until they puff and pop.

Chapter 11

Beans and Other Legumes

If you want to maintain a vibrant look of radiant health, then beans and lentils should be a frequent part of your diet. Beans contain protease inhibitors that interfere with cancer-causing enzymes, and also prevent the growth of cancer cells. Beans can also help lower serum cholesterol, triglycerides, and blood sugar. Beans are a power-packed, nutritious food.

—JOHN HEINERMAN
AUTHOR OF *HEINERMAN'S ENCYCLOPEDIA OF FRUITS, VEGETABLES, AND HERBS*

*b*eans, peas, and lentils are ancient foods—staples of every culture in which they grow, whether on plants, on climbing vines, or even on trees. Although most varieties originated in Africa, Asia, and the Middle East, nomadic tribes brought them overland into Europe and across the Bering Strait into the Americas, and they have been cultivated for thousands of years almost everywhere on earth. Lentils that predate the Esau story of the Old Testament are featured on the pyramids in Egypt, while others have been frozen in time by the cementlike lava of Vesuvius, preserved to this day in the ruins of Pompeii and Herculaneum.

Other archaeological evidence indicates that the Mexican Aztecs ate beans as far back as the tenth century, and that the Incas introduced them to South America. Much later and farther north, Native Americans on the east coast of what is today the United States taught the early settlers from Europe to plant corn and beans together so that the bean vines could climb the cornstalks and be supported by them. The natives also showed the settlers how to cook beans and corn together to create a dish called "muscicickquatash," which the settlers and their descendants transliterated to "succotash."

Legumes are grown and eaten on every continent except Antarctica. They are the second staple on earth, after rice, and dishes based on this PowerFood are signatures of a wide range of cultures: dal from India, hummus from the Middle East, refried beans or rice and beans from Latin America, black-eyed peas from the tribal lands of Native Americans.

Cheap, convenient, easy to find and keep, extremely versatile, beans and other legumes are basic, universal, and just a bit mundane—a poor-relation kind of food if ever there was one. Until recently.

The Power of This PowerFood

Beans and other legumes are well known as an excellent low-fat source of protein, fiber, iron, and calcium, containing almost as much protein as meat and dairy products, enough soluble and insoluble fiber to cleanse the blood of toxins and soothe the colon, enough iron and calcium to make legumes particularly recommended for women's blood and bone strength. Add to this the collection of phytochemicals now being attributed to legumes, and you have an extremely powerful fighter against disease and aging. In fact, in terms of value for money, beans and other legumes are one of the great health bargains around; for a minimal investment of money, time, and effort, you realize an extremely high return in nutrition and vitality. This may be why in recent years this PowerFood has begun to receive a great deal of good press.

The phytochemical stew in legumes includes linoleic and phytic acids, indoles, quercetin, coumarins, saponins, phytosterols, and lignans. All are cancer-blockers and antioxidants. In addition, the intense concentration of saponins in legumes is decisive; beyond their anticancer properties, there is evidence that these phytochemicals are potent blood-thinners and cholesterol-reducers. In fact, recent studies at universities in Kentucky and Minnesota and at a laboratory in the Netherlands have documented quite startling reductions in blood cholesterol as a direct result of adding legumes to the diet.

Such evidence confirms a highly proactive disease-fighting, anti-aging role for legumes. These are health benefits that add up to much more than a hill o' beans.

Colorful Cosmopolites

Beans and other legumes come in a wide variety of different forms and in a rainbow of colors and names. There are the kidney beans, split peas, lentils, and white beans popular in Europe; the chick-peas or garbanzos and favas of the Middle East and Africa; the adzuki beans that are staples of the markets in Japan and China.

Lima beans originated in the Andes Mountains, although today they also grow in California. Peas have become central to the cuisine of Italy. Black beans are favored in South America, and black-eyed peas, with their single black spot, are popular in the American South, especially in such spicy favorites as Hoppin' John. Pinto beans are the most popular bean in the United States and are a favorite in Mexican dishes and in Tex-Mex cuisine as well.

In many of these places and throughout their history, legumes have been eaten in combination with something else. Nutritionally speaking, that is because the protein in legumes is incomplete; it lacks one or more amino acids. By combining the legume with grains or with a small amount of an animal product like poultry, fish, meat, or a dairy product, one makes the protein complete.

In diets dominated by vegetables, or in parts of the world where eating animals is either prohibited by custom or prohibitively costly, the typical combination is legume and grain. Over time, this combination has been turned into a set of culinary classics: rice and beans, couscous and chick-peas, lentils and barley, and succotash. Such classics, and all the combinations that beans and other legumes can inspire, are an excellent guide to meal-planning when you're putting PowerFoods first.

Buying Beans and Other Legumes

Beans and other legumes come dried, canned, and cooked. They are widely available in supermarkets as well as in small groceries and health food stores. The canned product is an acceptable alternative to the dried if you are short on time, but it is wise to rinse the canned items to drain away some of the salt.

When buying dried legumes, look for whole, unbroken legumes with a color that is uniform throughout the package. Sniff the package; if there is a hint of sourness or rancidness, advise the store manager to check for freshness.

Dried beans and other legumes can be stored for almost a year at cool room temperature in tightly covered containers. Avoid leaving legumes in a warm, humid environment. Leftover cooked legumes should be stored in the refrigerator; they will keep for three to four days.

Washing and Sorting Beans and Other Legumes

Spread the legumes out on a light-colored cloth, sift them, or pick through them any way you like. You're looking for foreign matter—tiny pebbles, dust, debris, twigs, sand—and for damaged legumes or those shriveled with age. Be particularly careful with black beans and pinto beans; they're the worst offenders when it comes to damage and dirt. Once you've sorted through the legumes, put them in a strainer and rinse them thoroughly in cold water.

Soaking Beans and Other Legumes

All legumes *except* lentils and split peas, and, where clearly noted on the package, some newly available precooked versions of pinto beans and black beans must be soaked before cooking. Soaking is essential to keep cooking time reasonable and to take the fight out of the indigestible sugars that produce gas and bloating. You may see many different instructions about how to soak and how long to soak beans and other legumes. It really is not very complicated. There is slow soaking, and there is quick soaking.

For slow soaking, set the legumes in four times as much water and leave them overnight or for at least four to six hours. Another way to figure water-to-legume ratio is 10 cups of water per pound of beans or peas. For quick soaking, set the legumes in four times as much water (10 cups per pound), bring to a boil, and boil for two minutes. Then remove from the heat, cover the pot, and let stand for one hour.

Whichever method you use, skim off any items that may have floated to the top of the pot during soaking. Then pour off the soaking water. Drain thoroughly; the soaked legumes should be cooked in fresh water with as little trace as possible of the "dirt" you have just soaked off.

Cooking Beans and Other Legumes

The amount of water required for cooking will vary from legume to legume. In general, however, set the dried legumes in a large pot and add water to a level about two inches above the legumes. Bring to a boil. Then reduce the heat, skim the scum off the surface of the water, partially cover the pot, and simmer. Stir occasionally, doing so very gently so as not to break the skins of the legumes. For that reason also, make sure that the legumes are at a simmering, not rolling, boil. Over medium heat, it will take from one to three hours of cooking to achieve the right tenderness, again, depending on the variety of legume. For example, the colored and dappled legumes tend to take longer to cook; two exceptions are small white beans and garbanzos or chick-peas.

Cooking time also depends on the intended use of the legume you're cooking. If you're going to use the legumes in a salad, for example, and you therefore want them firm, or if you intend to use them in a casserole, soup, or stew where they will receive further cooking, go for a shorter cooking time. If, by contrast, you're going to mash or purée the legumes, choose the longer cooking times and leave them on the stove until soft. The following table shows typical cooking times for beans and other legumes.

Beans: Cooking Times and Proportions

Beans (1 cup)	Amount of Water	Cooking Time	Yield
Black beans	4 cups	1½ hours	2 cups
Black-eyed peas	3 cups	1 hour	2 cups
Garbanzos (chick-peas)	4 cups	3 hours	2 cups
Kidney beans	3 cups	1½ hours	2 cups
Lentils and split peas	3 cups	45 minutes	2½ cups
Limas	2 cups	1½ hours	1½ cups
Baby limas	2 cups	1½ hours	1½ cups
Pinto beans	3 cups	3 hours	2 cups
Red beans	3 cups	3 hours	2 cups
Small white beans (navy, etc.)	3 cups	2½ hours	2 cups

Another tip: Since acidic foods slow cooking, wait till the last moments of cooking legumes to add such ingredients as tomatoes or vinegar. The same goes for salt, which toughens the skin of the legumes and prolongs cooking time; add it dead last.

Crockpots and pressure cookers are both useful for cooking dried legumes. The crockpot provides slow, even heat and ensures thorough cooking. Boil the water first, then add the legumes and turn to a high setting; the legumes will cook as quickly as on the stove. A pressure cooker, by contrast, offers a fast, efficient way to cook beans, peas, and lentils. Follow the instructions supplied by the manufacturer of your particular pressure cooker.

You can also cook legumes in a microwave. Put them in a microwave-safe baking dish with twice their volume of water. Cook them at full power for eight to ten minutes or until they boil, then drop the power down to 50 percent and cook until tender, typically, another fifteen or twenty minutes. (Of course, if you are cooking fresh green legumes, cook, steam, stir-fry, microwave, or sauté them as you would any fresh vegetable.)

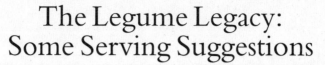

The Legume Legacy:
Some Serving Suggestions

The possibilities are endless. Legumes add texture and soak up flavor in salads, soups, stews, and sauces; in croquettes, casseroles, and curries; in purées, spreads, and dips; as a stuffing in the likes of eggplant or sweet peppers.

They combine wonderfully with the seasoning of such PowerFoods as garlic and company, mushrooms, all the crucifers and leafy greens, and, of course, whole grains—the classic marriages: lentil and barley soup; angel-hair pasta and dried peas; seven-bean salad; black beans and rice; Boston baked beans on brown bread; eggplant and chick-pea casserole; a legume sloppy joe on a roll.

Legumes really sit up and take notice when flavored with the spicy ingredients of such "hot" cuisines as the Mexican, Cajun, and Indian. Try them with coriander, cilantro, cumin, curry, and chiles. Mediterranean flavorings also delight. Try garlic, basil, sage, oregano, and rosemary.

Legumes are perfect in warm, comforting winter soups starring black beans, lentils, or split peas. And they work equally well in light summer fare when mixed with fresh greens and raw vegetables and herbs, as in lentils with arugula and watercress, cooked kidney beans with fresh green beans, black-eyed peas with carrots and celery.

Mashed-legume dips and spreads can replace cream cheese or sour cream. They work on sandwiches and are tasty side dishes. Kathie Swift suggests that many people who claim to dislike beans actually dislike their texture rather than their flavor; for these people, dips and spreads are the perfect way to get the power of beans.

Chapter 12

Soy and Soy Products

The strongest data we have about soy is in its effects on cardiovascular disease where you can see that it has biological impact. People with high cholesterol who add soy to their diet can actually lower the "bad" cholesterol and increase the "good." Many people in the world eat soy foods, and their risk of illnesses such as heart disease and cancer is much lower than in this country.

—DR. STEPHEN BARNES, UNIVERSITY OF ALABAMA

*a*mericans rarely see soy in its bean form. We're more familiar with roasted soy nuts as a snack; soy milk; tofu, tempeh, and miso soup served in Chinese and Japanese restaurants; or with soy flour or powdered protein used as an invisible ingredient in the "soyburgers" and soy ice creams that are just now moving out of health food stores into the mainstream. (Actually, we're perhaps *most* familiar with soy sauce and soy oil, but as processed foods, they have been robbed of their phytochemicals, so they do not qualify as PowerFoods.)

For another thing, we tend to think of soy as something foreign, exotic. It is true, of course, that the soybean (or soya bean, or soy pea) is indigenous to tropical and warm regions in China, Japan, and India, where it has been cultivated for at least five thousand years. But what is perhaps surprising is that the United States produces approximately half of the world's soybeans, which grow north of a line stretching west from Maryland to Kansas and picking up again west of the Rockies. Equally surprising is that we export a third of our soybean harvest, relegating most of the rest of it to industrial uses. It is only since the early 1980s that soy as a food has come into its own in the United States. And it is only in the 1990s that its power as a PowerFood has been demonstrated in the laboratory and in studies on human populations.

America's Soy Story

The short, stiff soy plant was first brought to this country from England in 1802. By 1920, the American soy harvest was one million bushels a year; by 1944, it was twelve million a year. Many of the uses to which the harvest was put were not edible, at least not by humans; the green crop was used for animal forage and hay, while by-products served as emulsifiers in glycerin, soaps, plastics, and food products.

Most of the crop that did go for human food was the export crop. In 1973, when President Richard Nixon ordered a temporary embargo on soybean exports, Japan, Korea, and other Asian countries felt the shock so profoundly that the White House bowed to pressure and lifted the ban after only five days. For Japan, even those five days had been traumatic; with the nation importing more than 90 percent of its soybeans from the United States for the bean curd, soy sauce, and cooking oil that are staples of the Japanese diet, the embargo had sent the price of soybeans in Japan soaring by 40 percent.

The Power of This PowerFood

The Japanese eat more soybean and soy products than any other single population on earth, an average of 23 pounds per person per year, versus perhaps two pounds of soy products eaten per American per year. The Japanese also have a longer life expectancy than any other population on earth. Japanese women suffer breast cancer only one-fourth as much as American women. The occurrence of colon cancer among Japanese is a third what it is among Americans. As reported in Chapter 2, when Japanese nationals move to the West and give up their soy-rich diet, their incidence of cancer shoots up. Such compelling evidence seems more than coincidental; at the very least, it suggests strongly that there's something in soy that strengthens cell resistance to free radicals and carcinogens.

Science has since confirmed the suppositions about soy's power. We have long known that soy is a rich source of protein; in fact, it is the only vegetable whose protein is complete. Now we know that it is loaded with phytochemicals—with isoflavones like genistein, cholesterol-lowering daidzein, protease inhibitors, phytic acids, saponins, phenolic acids, and intense concentrations of coumarins. This is a stew with potent properties as an antioxidant and with phytosterols that compete against the hormone-related cancers; it's a hormone-deflecting, tumor-suppressing, blood-thinning, virus-fighting, cholesterol-lowering warrior.

Genistein, for example, has been shown to thwart cancer at every stage of its development. It interferes with enzymes that "breed" cancer genes, cuts off the blood vessels that act as supply lines to developing cancers, stunts the growth of cancer cells. At the same time that genistein is stopping cancer cells, it also stops the growth of cells that can clog arteries, scavenging the free radicals that oxidize LDL cholesterol, the bad cholesterol. That makes soy an antidote to artery deterioration; some documented studies even conclude that it helps rejuvenate old arteries. A meta-analysis that reviewed the results of a number of studies confirmed that conclusion, finding an actual decrease in LDL, triglycerides, and overall total-cholesterol level among hundreds of people eating more than 47 grams of soy protein a day.

A protease inhibitor in soy, the Bowman-Birk inhibitor, is another powerful antioxidant against aging, various cancers, and other diseases. Daidzein manipulates estrogen to reduce the risk of breast cancer in both premenopausal and postmenopausal women.

No wonder soy-based formulas are now considered de rigueur for infants. In fact, some studies done on laboratory rats show that soybean intake early in life may serve as a lifelong dose of cancer-fighting agents, although such studies have yet to be undertaken on humans. In addition, soy protein does not provoke the allergic reactions seen with casein, the cow milk protein.

But What About the Taste?

With its nutritional value long established, the soybean has for some time enjoyed pride of place in the diet of the health-conscious. Now, as its supranutritional, phytochemical, disease-fighting power becomes increasingly evident, more and more medical experts and dietitians are recommending it. The problem is, however, that American taste buds to date just have not accepted soy or soy products.

One reason may be a misconception about the uses of soy. With its mild taste and porous consistency, soy takes on the flavors of the foods with which it is cooked. That is its strength—for both the by-the-book cook who can simply use it as a replacement in written recipes, or for the creative chef limited only by his or her imagination. And because soy foods come in so many different forms, you can get the benefits of this important PowerFood in everything from stir-fries to fruit shakes, from pancakes to pasta to pie, as a snack, in a salad, in an appetizer or a dessert.

Soy foods are typically divided into nonfermented and fermented categories. The nonfermented are the fresh green whole soybeans, whole dry soybeans, soy nuts (often roasted), soy flour, soy milk, and such soy milk products as tofu. The fermented category includes tempeh, miso, and the non-PowerFood soy sauces.

A new generation of soy foods is marketed as imitations of dairy and meat dishes: soy cheeses, soy burgers, soy sausages, soy yogurts, soy ice creams. For the most part, these foods are devised from textured soy protein—TSP—or they contain isolated soy protein, soy flour, or soy powder.

Using Your Bean

Soybeans are eaten both fresh and dried. The fresh beans are green, the dried range in color from tan to black. They are pea-sized and should be unbroken. Buy them in transparent packages so you can check for wholeness and for evenness of color. Stored in tightly covered jars and refrigerated, the dried beans should last six months.

Steamed fresh soybeans are a pure and simple main dish or accompaniment. Because the flavor tends to be bland, it is best to cook them with other, more vigorous ingredients and/or spices—for example, with such other PowerFoods as onions or rice or peppers, flavored with garlic. I adore them steamed in their pods and then popped out and eaten unadorned.

Dried soybeans should be prepared and cooked in the same way as any other bean (see Chapter 11). Cooking time tends to be long: three hours or more for two cups of dried soybeans, yielding four cups when done. Like any other bean, soy can be served as a main dish, side dish, accompaniment, and in soups or salads.

Roasted soybeans have become a snack food, packaged and sold like peanuts; the two are nutritionally similar, too, although their phytochemical content distinguishes them. These soy nuts add crunch to a salad, stir-fry, or side dish.

Miso

Miso is a paste made from fermented soybeans and a grain. It makes a wonderful base for flavoring soups, sauces, dressings, and stews; add it at the end of the cooking process because its complex flavor can change. A soothing cup of miso can be a comforting snack. A miso marinade is a top-notch addition to your usual favorite ingredients, and a miso spread adds a dab of PowerFood to your cracker, bread, or corn on the cob. Be careful, though: Part of miso's pungency is its saltiness; it is a high-sodium PowerFood.

Tofu

Probably the most famous soy product, tofu is equally well known as (soy)bean curd, and it has also been called "the cheese of Asia." In fact, it has the consistency of some cheeses and is made in a similar way. That is, a curdling agent, usually a natural sea salt called nigari, is added to soy milk; the resultant curd is pressed into cubes.

Precisely because of its very bland taste and porous consistency, tofu has great versatility, taking on the flavors of any foods with which it is cooked.

Tofu is now widely available in supermarkets across the country, sold as extrafirm, firm, soft, and silken. The extrafirm and firm are dense and solid; they hold up well in stir-fry dishes, soups, or on the grill—anytime, in fact, that you need the tofu to maintain its shape. The firm tofu tends to be higher in fat, although reduced-fat versions are now available.

The soft tofu results from a less aggressive pressing of the curd and is a good choice in recipes that call for blended tofu. Try it in salad dressings, shakes, pies, and cream soups.

Silken (or Japanese) tofu is made differently. The curds are not pressed but are allowed to set with the whey, resulting in a creamy, custardlike product that is actually firmer than "soft." Silken tofu works well in recipes calling for puréed or blended tofu.

It also works well in recipes that don't call for tofu at all. Nutritionist Kathie Swift feeds hordes of teenagers a macaroni and cheese dish that is actually made with tofu—although she doesn't tell that to the kids! The dish, which is particularly creamy and very tasty, is a cinch to make and takes no time at all:

While a pound of pasta is cooking, Kathie drains an 8-ounce carton of silken tofu, blends it in a blender until smooth and creamy, adds a cup of nonfat cottage or ricotta cheese, and blends until smooth. She then transfers the blend to a small saucepan, adds ½ cup of reduced-fat Cheddar cheese and ¼ cup of Parmesan or Romano cheese, and seasons with a dash of chili powder. Then she stirs in the drained pasta.

You will usually find tofu in the produce section of the market, although it may be in the dairy or deli sections—a hint of its versatility. It is sold in water-filled tubs, as aseptic brick packages, in vacuum packs, or already crumbled. Tofu is perishable unless aseptically packaged; it must be refrigerated and covered with water. If you buy it out of the tub, sniff to be sure it is not sour. If you buy it packaged, check for a freshness date. Once you have the tub-bought tofu home, or after you have opened the packaged tofu, it should be rinsed and covered with fresh water that is changed daily. Use any leftovers within a week. Silken tofu does not need refrigeration and lasts for about six months in the unopened package.

Tofu can also be frozen for up to five months. Drain the tofu and squeeze out all the excess water first, then seal the tofu in a tightly lidded container or freezer bag. As the tofu freezes, it will change color, taking on a caramel hue. The defrosted tofu retains this color, and it has a chewy texture that soaks up sauces and is great for grilling.

All tofu should be drained before eating. If it is not going to be cooked, it should be blanched: set it in a strainer and pour boiling water over it for about 20 seconds. When sautéing or stir-frying tofu, you can keep it from crumbling by shaking the pan or skillet rather than stirring the tofu itself.

Tofu's uses are almost limitless. Whip it into a tempting topping in place of whipped cream. Scramble it for an eggless morning wake-up call, or substitute two ounces of firm tofu for every egg in your egg salad recipe, or reach for the soyannaise instead of mayonnaise when making dips, spreads, or sandwich stuffers. Put it in the blender with fresh or frozen fruit and some honey for a creamy fruit shake. Break tradition by substituting it for cheese in lasagna. Try a dollop of tofu sour cream on your baked potato. Mash it and substitute it for cottage cheese or even chopped meat in your favorite recipe. And so on and on to the outer reaches of your culinary imagination.

Tempeh

A thin cake made from soybeans fermented with grains, tempeh originated in Indonesia. It has more protein than tofu, and it is considered to be far tastier. Cut into slices or patties, it makes a good substitute for beef in soups, chili, and casseroles; it's also a fine idea to coat it with barbecue sauce, grill it, and serve it on a toasted hamburger bun.

Soy Protein, Flour, and Milk

Isolated soy protein, in powder form, can be mixed into drinks, sauces, or pasta fillings, sprinkled over hot cereals, added to batters.

Textured soy protein (TSP), by contrast, mimics meat or poultry in texture but has a milder taste. With a little ingenuity, however, you can adapt your favorite recipes to take advantage of its power as a PowerFood. For example, use TSP instead of ground beef in chili; then just heat up the spicing to compensate for the milder flavor. In meat casseroles, let TSP replace half the animal protein, then adjust the seasoning accordingly.

Soy flour is a finely ground powder made from roasted soybeans, and soya powder is a finer ground, more flavorful form of this flour. Both are excellent in baking and for items like waffles and pancakes. Use ¼ cup of soy flour to one cup of all-purpose flour.

Soy milk is a noncurdled liquid extracted from cooked soy beans that are ground with water. It is sold in an assortment of flavors and is now available in a low-fat version. You can cook your grains or hot breakfast cereal in soy milk instead of water, and you can eat your cold cereal in it to boost the nutrient profile of your breakfast. Or, blend it with fruit into a fruit shake. Or, use it in baking recipes that call for milk. You can even mix it with fruit juice, chill it for an hour, and turn it into a fruit sorbet, cleansing the palate and charging up your well-being at the same time.

Chapter 13

Nuts and Seeds

Americans need to learn that fat, in itself, is not a nutritional evil, and that nuts are a healthy food. Nuts have virtually no chemical similarities to fatty animal foods and should not be grouped with them. Increasing evidence suggests that most nuts, and especially walnuts, will lower blood cholesterol when substituted for animal fats that are commonly used in the Western diet.

—DR. GARY FRASER,
DIRECTOR, CENTER FOR HEALTH RESEARCH
LOMA LINDA UNIVERSITY, LOMA LINDA, CA

*N*uts and seeds are the mythic diet of the so-called health food freak, and for that reason, they have typically been a target of derision. But don't be put off by the ridicule; these small packages contain a universe of disease-fighters and a world of well-being. When putting PowerFoods first, nuts and seeds become an important source of fat. Fat is a word freighted with unpleasant images for most of us, but like it or not, it is one of the basic nutrients of life—something we all need in some form or another. Nuts and seeds are a good form of fat.

In fact, the phrase "nuts and seeds" is something of a misnomer. That's because nuts for the most part are seeds. True nuts, like acorn, chestnut, and hazelnut, are the dry seeds—or strictly speaking, the one-seed fruits—of nonleguminous trees or shrubs, and they are encased in shells that don't open on their own.

In reality, however, just about any seed or fruit that contains an edible kernel inside a brittle covering is called a nut. It's true for

129

cashews, coconuts, pistachios, and walnuts. It's true for the elegant almond, which is actually the seed of a drupe—that is, of a stone fruit, a fleshy fruit with a single hard stone that encloses a seed. And perhaps the most famous nut of all, the peanut, is actually the pod of a pealike legume. Other edible seeds, like sunflower seeds or herb-produced sesame seeds, develop in softer fruits or pod capsules.

Whether we're talking about the bag of peanuts nervous fans devour at the ball park, or the sunflower seeds that are a hiker's favorite snack, nuts and seeds are a powerful PowerFood. That's because at the heart of the seed, carefully protected by that nutlike shell, is the seed's food storage tissue. It is a highly concentrated source of proteins and calories containing all the nutrients the plant embryo requires to grow and mature. What's good for plant sustenance is also healthy and beneficial for humans, which is why nuts and seeds serve as major sources of food for millions of people throughout the world.

Nuts and Seeds: History in a Nutshell

In fact, nuts and seeds have a very long history as staple foods. We tend to picture prehistoric man as a wanderer, scouring his environment for food, grazing on the nuts he could pull from shrubs and trees and on the seeds of plants blown by the wind. The picture is accurate. Nuts and seeds were part of our ancestors' diets from the moment the glaciers retreated and forests and plants began to grow in profusion. What's more, there is evidence that nut trees were cultivated as long ago as 10,000 B.C., which would make them one of the earliest examples of agriculture in human history.

Nuts and seeds play a role in the Book of Genesis in the Old Testament. When Jacob sends his sons to buy food in Egypt, he orders them to "take of the best products of the land . . . a little balm, and a little honey, spices and lotus, pistachio-nuts and almonds. . . ." And the Song of Songs speaks of going down "into the nut-garden, to look about among the plants of the valley. . . ."

Almonds, hazelnuts, chestnuts, pine nuts, and walnuts were favorite foods in ancient Rome. Nuts also served as baby rattles and as toys for Roman children. They were strewn on the floor at Roman weddings. And Roman women used nutshells to dye their hair.

In our own time, nuts are a mainstay of African cuisines. We know too that hickory nuts, chestnuts, pecans, black walnuts, beechnuts, and acorns were pervasive in the diet of Native Americans, and through them, these foods have entered the mainstream American diet. In fact, nuts and seeds are used routinely in many of the world's fine cuisines. Think of Chinese chicken with cashews, Italian pasta with pine nuts, or the elegant French dessert marrons glacés.

Many Uses in Many Places

Nuts and seeds aren't just edible nibbles, however. For centuries, they have been squeezed into pastes, pulverized into flours, pressed for oils, ground down and mixed with water for nourishing drinks.

Peanut oil and walnut oil are used in cooking. Walnut oil can clean and polish your wood furniture, jojoba nuts provide a lubricant for precision instruments, while tung oil features in paints and varnishes. The seeds of various plants provide the vegetable oils we cook with. Dill, mustard, pepper, and other seasonings come from seeds; beer, coffee, cocoa, and other drinks couldn't be made without seeds. Neither could detergents and soaps, livestock feed, some adhesives, and some explosives. Flax seed, increasingly being shown to be one of the most powerful of the PowerFoods, is pressed into linseed oil, which in turn creates linseed cakes for cattle fodder, and is also found in up-market hair styling gel—something to think about next time you're at the beauty salon. Meanwhile the fibers of the flax plant are made into fine papers, and the stems produce linen fabric, threads and cordage.

With all these uses, it's no wonder there's a growing demand for nuts and seeds. So while they grow wild just about everywhere on earth, produced by some three hundred species of shrubs and trees, this rising demand, coupled with rapid worldwide deforestation, has made nut-and-seed cultivation a profitable enterprise.

Today, about twenty-five kinds of nuts are raised as crops. Pecans are one of America's native nuts—essential for one of our greatest, richest desserts, pecan pie. California produces one-third of the world's supply of almonds and is the world's second largest producer of pistachios, which the state's growers first cultivated only in 1976. Pistachios originally come from the Middle East, where merchants dyed their beige shells red to hide blemishes. Hawaii ranks as the world's chief producer of macadamia nuts, originally from a tree indigenous to Australia. Walnuts and filberts are also significant U.S. nut crops.

Thanks to George Washington Carver, who showed farmers the many uses of the peanut, the American South—specifically Georgia—is the premier American producer of the peanut crop, although the United States ranks third, behind China and India, in growing peanuts. Under a variety of regional name changes—groundnuts, ground peas, Chinese nuts, and goobers—peanuts grace the sporting events and cocktail parties of Americans from sea to shining sea. In fact, we consume eight to nine pounds of peanuts per capita per year, most of it in the form of the whole peanut or peanut butter.

Seeds are harvested from plants grown around the world, then dried and packaged for commercial use. Flax, cultivated in China since perhaps 2000 B.C., is today grown in every region of the world, including the United States and Canada.

The tiny sesame seeds so basic to the cuisines of Africa, India, China, and the Middle East are supplied to U.S. buyers primarily by Latin American growers. Pumpkin and squash seeds are homegrown, as are the seeds of the sunflower, a plant native to North America. In fact, the sunflower is the state flower of Kansas, and if you drive across that state in late summer—or across any of the plains states as far up as North Dakota—you will see miles of bright yellow fields on the horizon. These are acres of sunflowers, standing up tall to face the sun, and soon to be harvested for their seeds to be used for poultry feed, oil, and snack foods.

The Power of This PowerFood

It is as a PowerFood that nuts and seeds are particularly useful. In fact, they are so nutritionally complete that a diet of nuts and seeds, rounded out by fruits and vegetables for vitamins A and C,

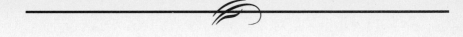

would be nutritionally complete. It might not be an entirely interesting diet, but it is entirely sufficient for well-being.

This is a PowerFood group rich in protein, fiber, vitamins, and minerals. As supranutritives, nuts and seeds are a top source of the antioxidant phytochemicals—lignans, monoterpenes, triterpenes and polyphenols—that block or slow the growth of protein-splitting enzymes.

Nuts and seeds contain the thiamine and folate essential to the nervous system. In fact, they contain prodigious amounts of all the B-complex vitamins. Their fiber and fatty acids lower cholesterol; walnuts, for example, have recently been shown to lower serum cholesterol and to favorably modify blood pressure in men. The calcium and potassium in nuts and seeds keep blood pressure steady; tiny sesame seeds contain almost ten times the calcium of an equal weight of milk.

Nuts and seeds have lecithin—good for reproductive and endocrine health and an important player in the health of the nerves. They are rich in iron, magnesium, and zinc—warriors against fatigue and stress. They're loaded with copper and selenium—antioxidants that gobble up free radicals bent on damaging your cell membranes and causing premature aging. In fact, the amount of these minerals in nuts and seeds is seven times the amount found in other types of fresh, minimally processed foods. Nuts and seeds are also rich in potassium, which works with other minerals to regulate heart rate and blood pressure. They also contain significant phosphorus, a building block of our bones and an essential generator of our metabolic energy supply.

But it's for their protein content that nuts and seeds are particularly valuable. The protein proportion of nuts weighs in at from 8 to 18 percent, while seeds derive 11 to 26 percent of their calories from protein. That's as much as the protein content of such legumes as beans. It's more than can be found in grains, cheese, eggs, and raisins. In fact, to get the amount of protein found in one pound of peanuts, you would have to drink nearly eight pints of milk. So nuts and seeds are a highly efficient source of needed protein. And this is plant protein, not the animal protein that in association with animal fat can contribute to the "bad" cholesterol.

Fat—And Essential

The other highly concentrated nutrient in nuts and seeds bears the unappealing name essential fatty acids, or EFA. Pay more attention to the word *essential* than to *fatty* or *acids*. EFAs are good fats, healing fats. They are just as important to health as proteins, minerals, and vitamins. In fact, EFAs used to be called Vitamin F. Just as with vitamins, deficiency of EFA is bad for our health.

Nutritionists are becoming increasingly alarmed about the excessive fear of fat fostered by the media. While consuming too much fat can of course lead to problems, so can eating too little fat. EFAs are essential for the stored energy they provide and because the body cannot make them. As a consequence, they must be obtained from food, and nuts and seeds—particularly in their natural, unprocessed form—are the best source of EFAs.

Of course, we can't ignore the "fatty" aspect of EFAs. On the one hand, they provide a large helping of energy in an efficient package. Nuts offer, on average, from about 140 to 165 calories per ounce; they derive between 70 and 97 percent of their calories from fat. (The delicious exception is chestnuts, which lower the curve at 70 calories per ounce, deriving only 8 percent of their calories from fat.)

On the other hand, for overfed Americans fighting the battle of the bulge, that level of calorie intake is a definite liability, even though the calories of nuts and seeds are inherently healthy. So consider this: If you were to substitute the "good" EFAs of nuts and seeds for the "bad" fats—butter, margarine, cheese, salad dressing, gravy, fast foods, for example—the overall nutritional content of your diet would be greatly improved with no increase in calorie intake. In other words, if you're going to eat fat, and we all must, eat it in the form of nuts and seeds, which do so much good in so many ways.

A Worthwhile Trade-off

In fact, in this trade-off—nuts and seeds instead of butter and gravy—the payback outweighs the liability. That's because the nutritional benefits of the EFAs in nuts and seeds are far greater than the risk of their calorie content.

Until recently, EFAs were considered useful simply because they were efficient storehouses of energy. But ongoing research has demonstrated that the monounsaturated and polyunsaturated fat of EFAs is required by the body for a variety of functions and is proactively useful against a variety of conditions.

In particular, the so-called omega–3 fatty acids attract oxygen and help keep it from wreaking havoc on body tissues. They form the membranes of our cells, control the way cholesterol works, lower triglycerides, reduce atherosclerosis, relieve arthritis by increasing the amount of anti-inflammatory prostaglandin in our bodies, and form part of the active tissue of the brain. These EFAs play key roles in regulating such biological functions as the cardiovascular system, the immune system, the digestive and reproductive systems. And by helping achieve the proper balance of calcium in our cellular structure, the omega–3 fatty acids also help prevent osteoporosis.

The omega–3 fatty acids are the major ingredients in fish-oil supplements touted as fighting coronary heart disease and relieving arthritis. You can get these cholesterol and inflammation reducers in adequate doses in nuts and seeds, but especially in flax seed, available in health and specialty stores as a snack or cereal. Indeed, as this ancient food gets a fresh look through a very contemporary lens, it appears to have more and more benefits.

The EFAs of nuts and seeds also contain liberal amounts of omega–6 or linoleic acid—the most essential of the essential fatty acids, the healthy fat that actually lowers blood cholesterol levels. Along with zinc, which is also present in seeds and nuts, linoleic acid has also been shown to be important in maintaining clear skin. It may help relieve asthma, mitigate the effects of premenstrual syndrome, even reduce the harshness of alcohol addiction withdrawal.

Contemporary research confirms that EFAs are not biologically active on their own. Rather, they must undergo a complicated biochemical conversion within the body. That means they're most effective when taken as part of a kaleidoscopic diet—a further argument, if any were needed, for balance, variety, and moderation as a pathway to well-being.

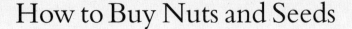

How to Buy Nuts and Seeds

We no longer have to graze for nuts and seeds as our ancestors did; they're available—mostly in the shelled variety—at the nearest supermarket, corner store, or health food shop. What's more, they come in vacuum-sealed cans, boxes, bags, or jars; whole, chopped, or slivered; shelled or unshelled; raw, dry, or roasted—even spiced.

Whatever variant you buy, be sure to check the freshness date on the package. Fresh nuts in the shell are available seasonally, typically in the fall and early winter. Look for chestnuts from September through March. Coconuts, the biggest plant seeds on earth, are best from October to December.

Note that peanuts are highly susceptible to a mold known as aflatoxin, a poison that can cause liver cancer. The aflatoxin fungus grows under hot and humid conditions, but careful harvesting, quick drying, and controlled storage prevent its growth, and the peanut industry has demonstrated great care in carrying out its responsibilities on this issue. Buy vacuum-packed or factory-packaged nuts and seeds with confidence.

When you do buy packaged nuts and seeds, get them in clear packages so you can see what you're getting. Avoid any that look limp. If selecting from bins, heft a few items in turn. Each should feel heavy, substantial. Check for crispness and definitely avoid any musty or rancid odor. If you're buying nuts in the shell, shake a few individual nuts to make sure the kernel doesn't rattle; if it does, the nut may be dry. When you lift a coconut, you want to feel a solid weight; shake it and listen: It should be full of liquid.

Seeds are routinely found packaged or in open bins in health food stores. Sunflower seeds and sesame seeds, however, have made their way into mainstream grocery stores and supermarkets, and flax seed packages will probably follow in due time.

An excellent way to obtain pumpkin seeds is to harvest your Halloween jack-o-lantern. Instead of discarding the seeds—which, by the way, are treasure-houses of zinc—fry them or roast them for a great garnish or savory snack.

Squirreling Away Nuts and Seeds: Storage and Preparation

Whole nuts keep better than pieces; unprocessed, unroasted, and/or unsalted keep better than processed; and nuts in the shell keep better than shelled (the shells, protecting against light and heat, prevent rancidity). Shelled nuts kept in tightly closed containers—either the original jar, freezer bags, or plastic bowls with sealing tops—will keep for up to four months. Refrigerated, they'll keep even longer. In the freezer, they'll stay good for up to a year. What's more, frozen nuts don't have to be thawed for cooking purposes, although if you're going to munch, toast briefly before serving, for extra flavor.

The first step in preparation is to crack the shells. On soft shells like peanuts, bare hands will do, but for walnuts and the like, you'll need a nutcracker. Actually, a hammer works just as well; stand the nut on end, hold it at the seam, and strike the top. Really hard nuts—Brazil nuts, for example—are easier to get to if they have been frozen first. Another useful tool is a nutpick; use it to extract absolutely every bit of the kernel, especially with walnuts and delicious black walnuts.

Most nuts and seeds taste better if they're toasted, roasted, or blanched, but they're also delicious, and at their nutritional best, when eaten raw. Roasting actually differs from toasting in that the process officially requires added fat, but for our purposes, we'll consider roasting and toasting equivalent. In any event, the process serves to burnish the flavor of nuts and seeds and to enhance their crispness as an accompaniment.

Preparing Nuts

Spread shelled nuts or seeds in a single layer on a greased pan or skillet. Bake in a 350°F. oven until lightly browned, anywhere from 10 to 20 minutes. In a microwave, use a paper plate, and cook for one and a half minutes at 100 percent power, stir again, let stand for a minute, and zap for another one and a half minutes. On top of the stove, toast the nuts or seeds in a skillet over medium heat until golden brown, about three to five minutes for seeds, five to ten for nuts.

Chestnuts can be roasted/toasted in the oven. Incise an X in the flat side of each shell, place the chestnuts in a shallow pan, cover tightly with foil, and cook for half an hour at 450°F. Shake the pan now and again while the chestnuts are roasting. Or, you can do as the song says and roast chestnuts over an open fire. If you don't have a fireplace grill—or actual chestnut roaster, available in some kitchen supply stores—wrap the chestnuts in heavy-duty foil and punch a few air-holes in the foil. Placed about five inches above the flame, the chest-nuts will take about 15 to 20 minutes to roast, depending on the heat of your fire.

The easiest way to blanch nuts with thin inner skins is to pour boiling water over the shelled nuts. Then drain the nuts, slide the skins off, and dry them on a paper towel. Or, sliver or slice the still warm nuts with a thick knife. Blanching is particularly recommended for walnuts and almonds, which often taste slightly bitter because of the tannic acid in their skins.

To grind nuts, the best tool is a grater or nut mill. Chop nuts, half a cup at a time, in a high-speed blender. To make your own nut butter, add a handful of nuts at a time to a blender or processor until the contents form a paste. To make the "chunky" variety, chop some additional nuts and fold them into the nut butter.

Some Nutty Ideas

One of the great strengths of nuts and seeds as a PowerFood is their versatility. They add crunch as well as flavor to almost all of your favorite foods. Put them in sauces; change them into butter pastes; sprinkle them on salads and desserts; garnish a stir-fry or soup with them; bake them in breads (but don't use sunflower seeds in quick bread recipes requiring baking soda unless you also add an acid ingre-dient or some honey; otherwise, the bread will be green—harmless, but not pretty). And of course, nuts and seeds are the quintessential healthy snack (in moderation).

My own favorites among the nuts are almonds and walnuts. My

PowerFoods

preferred seeds are sesame and flax. The nuts keep my cholesterol down; the seeds provide bone-strengthening calcium and protein, so important for women in particular. Both nuts and seeds provide a delicious source of steady energy. Moreover, their versatility in the kitchen is unequaled. They add substance to fruit salads, pep up ordinary potato salad or cole slaw, turn an everyday vegetable stir-fry into a dish fit for company, and make the perfect dessert topping—there is nothing like slivered almonds to perk up your rice pudding or add a touch of elegance to a fruit compote. I find that if I have a good supply of these essentials in the house, I can handle everything from quick snacks to company for dinner.

As a garnish, nuts and seeds add taste and crunch to bland, smooth foods. Chopped nuts and whole seeds improve breakfast cereals, vegetable and fruit platters, pasta, salads. A variation on the traditional potato salad, adding walnuts, parsely, and mustard vinaigrette, creates a new taste treat. Substitute chopped nuts for croutons as a topping for soups and salads.

Walnuts, almonds, pistachios, and sunflower seeds are particularly good in grain stuffings for vegetables, in rice pilaf or risotto, or tossed into pasta. Convert your child's PB and J into a sandwich made of homemade peanut or almond butter—a moderate amount—and fresh apple or banana slices. Make nut loaf instead of meat loaf for more protein, more iron, more vitamin E, and more fiber than the latter can come close to providing.

Whenever a recipe calls for nuts or seeds, use small amounts, put them on top where they will show, and leave some in bigger pieces— a real treat when you land one. Incorporate chopped nuts or seeds in bread or muffin batters. Make your own trail mix by combining pumpkin and sunflower seeds and chopped nuts with dried fruits. Combine almonds, dates, and water into an almond milk, a traditional "brain food." Sprinkle nuts on baked fruits or fruit crisps for dessert. Turn blanched almonds into either almond paste or marzipan, two delicious and typically expensive delicacies—and gain a reputation as an inventive home cook.

The Top Ten PowerFoods

PowerFood	Phytochemicals	Benefits
Red, yellow, and orange fruits	Carotenoids, terpenes, flavonoids, coumarins, vitamin C, boron, fiber	Antioxidants, protect vision, prevent degenerative disease (such as arthritis, heart disease, diabetes).
Red, yellow, and orange vegetables	Carotenoids, flavonoids, capsaicin, vitamin C, vitamin E, fiber	Antioxidants, protect vision, prevent degenerative disease (such as arthritis, heart disease, diabetes).
Cruciferous and leafy green vegetables	Indoles, carotenoids, isothiocyanates, vitamin C, vitamin E, magnesium, calcium, iron, fiber	Neutralize free radicals, stimulate anticancer enzymes, useful in asthma, knock harmful hormones off track.
Mushrooms	Lentinan, B vitamins, copper, fiber	Boost immune system, antiviral, antitumor, prevent abnormal clotting.
Sea vegetables	Carotenoids, vitamin C, calcium, iodine, fiber	Promote strong bones, boost metabolism, minimize heavy metal toxicity.
Garlic and company	Organosulfur compounds, allicin, quercetin, selenium, phosphorus, iron, potassium, fiber	Lower LDL cholesterol, fight infections, fight cancer, boost heart health, anti-inflammatory.
Whole grains	Lignans, phenolic acids, phytosterols, B vitamins, vitamin E, magnesium, chromium, fiber	Lower cholesterol, help prevent colon cancer, aid in elimination, improve insulin sensitivity, energy source.

PowerFood	Phytochemicals	Benefits
Beans and other legumes	Phytosterols, isoflavones, protease inhibitors, saponins, B vitamins, calcium, fiber	Lower LDL cholesterol, anticancer enzymes, alter harmful hormone pathways, aid elimination, promote healthy digestive system.
Soy and soy products	Flavonoids, phytosterols, saponins, protease inhibitors, fiber	Lower heart disease risk, fight cancer (especially hormone-related cancers in prostate, breast, and ovaries), useful in diabetes, may reduce menopause symptoms.
Nuts and seeds	Lignans, B vitamins, vitamin E, copper, selenium, calcium, essential fatty acids, fiber	Boost immune system, lower cholesterol, aid elimination, anti-inflammatory, stimulate enzymes that detoxify carcinogens.

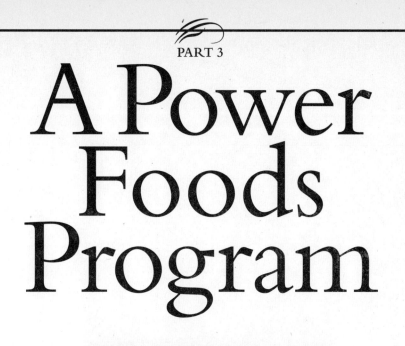

PART 3

A Power Foods Program

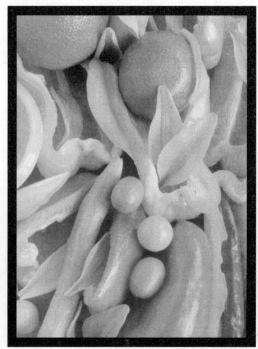

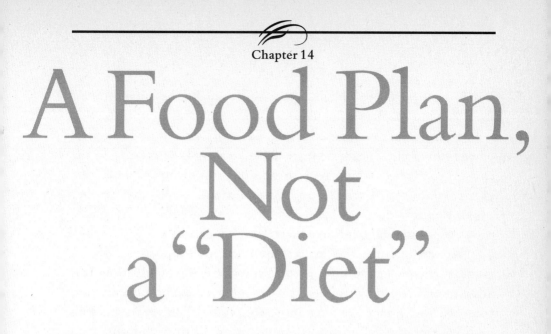

Chapter 14

A Food Plan, Not a "Diet"

Until one is committed, there is hesitancy, the chance to draw back, always ineffectiveness . . . The moment one definitely commits oneself, then Providence moves too. All sorts of things occur to help one that would never otherwise have occurred . . . Whatever you can do, or dream you can, begin it. Boldness has genius, power, and magic in it. Begin it now.

—JOHANN WOLFGANG VON GOETHE

*t*he PowerFoods Program has three components:

○ First, a food plan—a comprehensive system for eating that puts PowerFoods first, whether your goal is all-around well-being, weight loss, or building bulwarks against specific ailments or disorders;

○ Second, changed behavior—ensuring that you continue to put PowerFoods first wherever you are, whatever the situation;

○ Third, physical activity—the absolute essential for health and well-being for a lifetime.

It takes commitment to undertake the PowerFoods Program, but to paraphrase the quote by Goethe that opens this chapter, there is no way to begin except to begin. Once you've made the commitment, the following chapters will guide you along the path.

The program's premise is simple: Eat more PowerFoods, and less of everything else. Ideally, you are already eating PowerFoods, so the change you'll be making will be one of proportions. You will eat greater amounts of fruits and vegetables and beans, and smaller amounts of low-nutrition foods, whether high-fat villains like cheese and steak, or low-fat nerds like pretzels and pasta.

Precisely because it's a matter of choice and proportion, this is a program anyone can follow anytime, anywhere, in any situation. It is not a diet. If you stray from the program for a meal or a day or two, you have not undone the program's good; you can simply begin again with your next meal. Instead of deprivation, calorie-counting, and "nutritional supplements," the PowerFoods program relies on balance, variety, moderation. It asks you to appreciate, not enumerate, the diversity of nature's bounty, and to enjoy, not avoid, the pleasures of food that looks good and tastes good. But it also asks that you feed not just your mouth and stomach but the rest of your body as well—cells and organs, tissues and bones, energy level and all-around well-being.

Starting Point

In trying to get from where you are to where you want to be, the first step is to map out your eating habits. Start by keeping a food diary for three days; you'll find a sample diary worksheet at the end of this chapter. The three days need not be consecutive; in fact, it's a good idea to make one of the days Saturday or Sunday.

Be specific and absolutely honest in recording what you eat. Write down what you've eaten as soon as you've eaten it. Research on recall just hours after eating shows that most people remember only about 70 percent of what they've actually eaten. Give details; a turkey sandwich may also contain such PowerFoods as tomato, lettuce, onion, and whole grain bread, or it may simply be an excess of turkey on white bread with mayonnaise.

Once you have completed a three-day food diary, sit down with the three worksheets, take a colored marker, and highlight the

PowerFoods you ate during the course of those three days. The result is a picture of both your current PowerFood intake and your intake of everything else, a picture that should point the way toward your own personal prescription for eating more PowerFoods (and a variety of them) and less of everything else.

Is it possible to have a food diary with no highlights at all? Unfortunately, it is. Imagine a day that starts with a doughnut and coffee for breakfast, moves on to lunch of a cheeseburger with French fries and a soda, proceeds to a dinner of take-out spareribs and chips, and ends with a late evening snack of ice cream and cookies. In my experience as a physician, I have seen all too many such nutrition lapses, and I have seen patients who repeat their mistakes day after day. If you are such an eater, take heart—the only direction you have to go is up.

For most people, the path to becoming a PowerFoods eater is not so steep. For example, if your highlighted food diary shows that you eat about 30 percent PowerFoods and 70 percent everything else, you have some distance to travel to put PowerFoods first in your diet. On the other hand, if your diary shows just the opposite—70 percent PowerFoods and 30 percent everything else—you're well on your way, although you still want to improve. How to go about it?

The answer is to follow a food plan. A food plan is not a diet as we know it. The PowerFoods plan does not tell you precisely what to eat three times a day for a specific number of days. It offers guidelines and strategies that aim to help, not punish, you as you work toward your goal. Its aim is to bolster your self-esteem, increase your energy, and strengthen your immune system.

Your Personal PowerFoods Plan: The Basic Formula

A food plan is your personal prescription for putting PowerFoods first. To get it underway, spend a moment articulating the outcome you're hoping for. Are you doing this as a way to provide more nutritious eating for yourself, and at the same time to serve as a role model for your children? Is it a means to increase your energy level? Has a significant milestone made you more health-conscious—i.e., did you just turn forty? are you about to be fifty? Does a family history of heart disease, diabetes, or cancer have you scared? Do you want to improve your appearance—body shape, skin tone, hair health, nails? Perhaps you're following up on last New Year's resolution to get healthy once and for all.

For any of these reasons, or perhaps all of them at once, here's a basic formula for eating more PowerFoods and less of everything else, without worrying about calorie-counting or gram-counting:

○ **Have one fruit at each meal or snack.**
○ **Have a vegetable at lunch, dinner, and as a snack—and remember for variety to include mushrooms, sea vegetables, onions, and garlic along with all the wonderful green, red, yellow, and orange vegetables.**
○ **Eat a whole grain food or starchy vegetable at every meal.**
○ **Have at least one serving of legumes—all varieties of peas and beans, including the soybean—at lunch and/or dinner.**
○ **Garnish soups, stews, and salads with nuts and seeds, or have them, in moderation, as a snack.**

Your adaptation of this basic formula constitutes your personal PowerFoods plan. Here's how the formula looks meal by meal.

Ideal PowerFoods Plan

Breakfast	fruit		grain		
Snack			grain		
Lunch	fruit	vegetable	grain	legume or protein	seeds
Snack			grain		nuts
Dinner		vegetable	grain	legume or protein	
Snack	fruit		grain		

PowerFoods

Consider breakfast, for example. The plan suggests a fruit and a grain. The choices for each PowerFood are numerous, to say the least. The possible combinations are endless. To get some ideas, just look at our PowerFoods Menu Plan on pages 152–155. You are limited only by your own imagination, by what you like, and by what's available at the market. The same is true of the other two meals and the snacks, and the result is the same: There is no loss of taste variety when you create your personal PowerFoods plan from this basic formula.

A Nutrition Chart for Your PowerFoods Plan

While no one food plan fits all, all our food plans focus on low-fat PowerFoods that are rich in phytochemicals, vitamins, minerals, and fiber. Nutrition labels, however, don't list phytochemicals—not yet, anyway—so you may want to copy this book's Top Ten PowerFoods table (pages 140–141) and keep it with you when you shop for food, or even when you go out to a restaurant.

All PowerFoods are of course sources of important vitamins and minerals, but it may help to know which foods to look for to add particular vitamins and minerals to your diet. Refer to the "Nutrient-Rich Foods" chart to ensure you get adequate vitamins and minerals in your PowerFoods diet.

Nutrient-Rich Foods

Thiamine (Vitamin B1)	Pyridoxine (Vitamin B6)	Vitamin A
Brewer's yeast	Bananas	Sweet potatoes
Sunflower seeds	Whole grains	Carrots
Dried beans	Wheat germ	Kale
Salmon	Brown rice	Spinach
Brown rice	Dried beans	Cantaloupe
Whole grains	Chicken	Broccoli
	Salmon	Winter squash
		Apricots

(continued)

Riboflavin (Vitamin B2)

Broccoli
Spinach
Brewer's yeast
Soybeans
Eggs
Whole grains

Vitamin B12

Salmon
Milk
Eggs
Tofu
Chicken
Shellfish

Vitamin C

Citrus fruits
Green peppers
Brussels sprouts
Broccoli
Cantaloupe
Strawberries
Potatoes
Tomatoes

Niacin (Vitamin B3)

Peanuts
White potato
Brewer's yeast
Brown rice
Salmon
Tuna

Folacin

Broccoli
Brewer's yeast
Spinach
Fresh orange juice
Romaine lettuce
Brussels sprouts
Dried beans

Zinc

Pumpkin seeds
Peanuts
Oatmeal
Dried beans
Poultry, dark meat

Calcium

Broccoli
Kale
Almonds
Sesame seeds
Figs
Apricots
Yogurt
Milk, low-fat
Sardines
Salmon
Greens
Tofu
Blackstrap molasses

Iron

Broccoli
Spinach
Lean beef
Dried beans
Prunes
Raisins
Turkey, dark meat
Blackstrap molasses
Brewer's yeast

Potassium

Potatoes
Avocado
Dried fruits
Dried beans
Oranges
Bananas
Winter squash
Tomatoes
Sardines
Flounder

In addition to vitamins and minerals, fiber is essential for lowering cholesterol, and research shows that it plays a role in preventing colon cancer. Although fiber is nonnutritive for humans, it is the preferred food of the friendly bacteria that live in our gastrointestinal tracts. Those bacteria in turn produce the short-chain fatty acids that nourish the cells lining our large intestine or colon. The importance of fiber means that it should be a regular part of every diet. Look for such important high-fiber PowerFoods as the foods shown in the following chart.

Important Fiber Foods

Grains
Barley
40 percent bran flakes
Brown rice
Cracked wheat bread
Oatmeal bread
Oatmeal or rolled oats
White popcorn (plain), popped
Shredded wheat

Fruits
Apples
Apricots
Cantaloupe
Figs
Grapefruit
Grapes
Oranges
Peaches
Prunes
Raisins
Raspberries

Nuts and Seeds
Almonds
Pumpkin seeds
Sesame seeds
Sunflower seeds
Walnuts

Legumes
Dried beans
   Great Northern
   Kidney
   Lima
   Navy
Dried peas
Lentils
Soybeans

Vegetables
Broccoli
Brussels sprouts
Cabbage
Carrots
Cauliflower
Mushrooms
Onions
Potatoes
Sea Vegetables
   Dulse
   Nori
   Wakame
Spinach
Squash

A PowerFoods Menu Plan

      Perhaps the best tool for undertaking a PowerFoods program is menu planning. The recipes that constitute Part 4 of this book all put PowerFoods first. They all ensure that you're eating more PowerFoods and less of everything else. They are versatile enough to suit any occasion, from afternoon tea on Thursday to a company dinner on Friday night to a picnic lunch on Saturday and a Sunday brunch, not to mention everyday eating. Here's a week's worth of menus that embody the credo of balance, variety, and moderation and that sample foods from all the PowerFood groups. Follow this plan, modify it, adjust it to your personal tastes, and you are automatically undertaking your personal PowerFoods program.

Sunday

Brunch

> Fruit Compote
> Papaya Fig Bruschetta
> Scrambled Tofu Fiesta
> Stuffed Mushrooms
> Citrus Asparagus Salad
> Orange and Fig Muffins
> Blueberry Loaf

Supper

> Minestrone
> Barry Bread
> Arugula, Radicchio, and Endive Salad
> Baked Apples with Cherries and Walnuts

Monday

Breakfast

> Tropical Fruit Cup
> Buckwheat Muffins
> Peach Butter

Lunch

Asian Noodle Salad
Marinated Wakame and Zucchini Sticks
Blackberry Kanten

Dinner

Cream of Mushroom Soup
Baked Halibut with Herb Bread Crumb Topping
Stir-fried Broccoli
Greek Tabbouleh Salad
Apple Cranberry Crisp

Tuesday

Breakfast

Pineapple Banana Shake
Bran Muffins

Lunch

Kale Soup
Four-bean Salad
Steamed Cauliflower with Chive Butter
Sweet Potato Muffins

Dinner

Pasta with Zucchini Sauce
Fresh Tomatoes with Mozzarella
Cucumber Salad
Cantaloupe Sorbet

Wednesday

Breakfast

Danish Applesauce
Pumpkin Bread

Lunch

Barbecue Bean Soup

Spinach Hummus

Roasted Red Peppers and Brussels Sprouts

Dinner

Root Vegetables and Lamb Stew

Arugula and Radicchio Salad with Sherry Vinaigrette

Peach Frisée

Thursday

Breakfast

Fresh Melon Compote

Rice Flour Pancakes

Raspberry Sauce

Lunch

Stuffed Tomatoes with Rice and Pecans

Warm Cucumber Salad

Afternoon Tea

Sweet Potato Gingerbread

Banana Cherry Nut Bread

Fresh Strawberries Chantilly

Supper

Baked Papaya Skewers with Curry Sauce

Lemon-zested Couscous Dinner Salad

Friday

Breakfast

Gingered Tangerines with Mint

Grape-Nuts Muffins

Lunch

Mango and Watercress Salad with Marinated Chicken

Sweet and Spiced Baby Carrots

Cold Blueberry Soup

Company Dinner

Grilled Tuna Steaks with Ginger Mayonnaise

Citrus Butternut Squash

Spinach and Mushroom Stir-Fry

Hijiki Tossed Salad

Apricot Poppy Seed Cake

Saturday

Breakfast

Sweet Potato Pancakes

Cranberry Chutney

Picnic Lunch

Vegetable Chili

Corn Bread

Sweet Potato Chips

Apple Coleslaw

Potatoes with Vegetable Salsa

Beets with Tarragon

Caesar Salad

Tofu Brownies

Supper

Carrot Soup

Barley Risotto

Braised Swiss Chard

Baked Quince

My Three-Day Food Diary

Day 1   **Date**

Food Item and Method of Preparation	Amount Eaten

Day 2   Date

Food Item and Method of Preparation	Amount Eaten

Day 3   Date

Food Item and Method of Preparation	Amount Eaten

Chapter 15

The PowerFoods Weight-Loss Formula

I can resist everything, except temptation.
—OSCAR WILDE, *LADY WINDERMERE'S FAN*

Things do not change; we change.
—HENRY DAVID THOREAU, *WALDEN*

*Y*ou'll probably find that following a PowerFoods plan automatically leads to weight loss without dieting, without deprivation, and without cravings. Your new way of eating will simply make you feel more energetic and therefore more active—and suddenly, those last ten pounds that would never budge are just gone.

But suppose weight loss is the outcome you're hoping for in starting a PowerFoods program. To create such a weight loss plan, you may need to do something I usually oppose vigorously—that is, count what you eat. Indeed, throughout this book, the idea of *dimensioning* food—counting calories, weighing and measuring portions—has been scrupulously avoided. Such a practice teaches you how to count; it does not instill the basics of a way of eating. But *some* counting will be necessary to get the momentum going in your personal PowerFoods weight loss plan. The reason is simple: If you are going to lose weight by eating more PowerFoods and less of everything else, you will need to count both PowerFoods and everything else until you've achieved the balance that is right for you, and until choosing a variety of PowerFoods in moderation becomes second nature.

Calories: Your Own Daily Requirement

The first step toward weight loss is to determine your personal calorie level—that is, what your daily calorie intake *ought to be*. (Remember that a calorie is a measure of heat that is contained in food and released upon oxidation by the body; it's a serving of energy-producing potential.) Obviously, your body requires some number of calories in order to maintain vital functions, even when at rest. In fact, "at rest" is a relative term, for when you're at rest, your heart is beating, your lungs are expanding and contracting with each breath, your liver is making enzymes, your kidneys are cleansing the blood flowing throughout your circulatory system. In short, there's a lot going on in a body at rest, a level of activity that's been estimated at one billion biochemical reactions per second. These reactions require energy, and we call this level of energy, measured in calories, the basal metabolic rate—BMR.

The rule of thumb is that a twenty-year-old woman needs a daily calorie amount that is eleven times her body weight and a twenty-year-old man needs a level that is twelve times his body weight just to maintain basal metabolic functions. If the twenty-year-old woman weighed 140 pounds, her BMR would therefore be 1540 (140 × 11); if the twenty-year-old man weighed 170, he would need 2040 (170 × 12). To begin to figure out your BMR, if you're a woman, multiply your current weight by eleven; if you're a man, multiply your current weight by twelve. Calculate your BMR.

But gender isn't the only factor that affects BMR. So does age: The older you are, the lower your BMR is likely to be. That's because most people lose muscle mass and gain fat as they age, and since muscle is our calorie-burning tissue, muscle loss slows our metabolic rate. So right off the bat, subtract 2 percent from the above number for each decade you claim past the age of twenty. For example, our 140-pound woman at age 50 would have a BMR of 1540 minus 6 percent (2 percent × 3): 1448. Calculate your age-adjusted BMR.

Remember: This age-adjusted number you have calculated is still the BMR—the required daily calorie intake for maintaining vital functions while at rest. The fact is, however, that no one is at rest twenty-four hours a day. Even the biggest couch potato gets up in the morning, brushes her teeth, gets dressed, and moves around to some extent. So in general, even for the most sedentary lifestyle, we can add back 10 percent of the adjusted BMR just for being up and about. That means that our fifty-year-old, inactive, 140-pound woman with the age-adjusted BMR of 1448 would actually need a minimum daily intake of 1593 calories (1448 + 145) to meet her basic needs, and this amount of calories will result in weight loss over time, especially if she increases her activity level. So increase your age-adjusted BMR by 10 percent to determine your needed daily intake of calories. Calculate your personal daily calorie intake.

Remember, your BMR is an amount calculated to meet your body's most basic needs at its least active. To try to lose weight with fewer calories will lead to failure; on the other hand, to be able to eat more food and still lose weight means you must increase your activity. The more active you are, the more calories you burn and the more you can eat and still lose weight. As will be discussed in greater detail in Chapter 18, activities can range from light work like house cleaning, at about 180 calories per hour, to a moderate exercise like canoeing at 230 calories per hour, to such vigorous pursuits as cycling (650 calories per hour), running (800 calories per hour), and cross-country skiing (1200 calories per hour). That means an hour of exercise can equal anywhere from a tenth to a third to three-fourths to a whole day's worth of food just for having fun outdoors on a beautiful day. The bottom line is to increase your activity and adjust your daily calorie intake appropriately. Just remember: Eat more PowerFoods and less of everything else. Then reap the benefits. In the meantime, hold on to your adjusted BMR figure; we'll come back to it in a minute.

Your Personal PowerFoods Weight Loss Plan

The creation of your personal PowerFoods plan rests on the basic assumption that an individual's daily diet comprises (and should comprise) something from each of the following six categories of food:

○ **fruit**
○ **vegetables**
○ **complex carbohydrates**
○ **proteins**
○ **fats**
○ **dairy and nondairy**

When your daily diet includes foods from all of these categories, you are ensuring that you get all needed vitamins, minerals, and phytochemicals in a varied, balanced diet of moderate portions.

Of course, you are also putting PowerFoods first, as all ten PowerFoods fit into those six categories. The fruit category contains all red, yellow, and orange fruits. As for the berries, they belong to the red fruit category; although they may look blue or black, they all share the phytochemical profile of the red fruits and are very potent PowerFoods. Vegetables include the red, yellow, and orange vegetables, the crucifers and leafy greens, mushrooms, sea vegetables, and garlic and company. Complex carbohydrates are the whole grains, starchy vegetables, and the legumes—beans, peas, and soy. Fats include nuts, seeds, and the high-fat vegetables such as olives and avocados, not to mention plant-based oils.

Our only departure from PowerFoods is the protein and dairy categories, and they deviate only partially. Protein, for example, is in legumes and whole grains as well as lean meat, chicken, and fish. And while dairy includes low-fat milk, low-fat yogurt, and low-fat cheese, nondairy includes milk and cheese products made from soy, rice, oats, almonds, and sesame seeds. This means that vegetarians who do not wish to eat any animal products can still fulfill their requirements for protein and for the vitamins and nutrients most readily found in dairy foods.

Meat, chicken, fish, and dairy foods are included in the PowerFoods program because it would be unrealistic *not* to include them; they are, after all, elementary aspects of the American diet. Life need not be meatless and dairyless to be healthy. Just check our PowerFoods recipes, with the likes of Grilled Tuna Steaks with Ginger Mayonnaise or Cream of Mushroom Soup or Root Vegetables and Lamb Stew or Fresh Tomatoes with Mozzarella.

So we start our PowerFoods weight loss plan with the commitment to eat these six categories of food every day. How much of each every day? First, go back to your BMR adjusted for age and minimal activity.

We'll count in servings, and the number of servings will vary depending on the individual's desired daily calorie intake, as shown in the following table, where each column represents a hundred-calorie range.

Servings of Food for Daily Calorie Intake

Calories	1400	1500	1600	1700	1800	1900	2000
Fruits	4	4	4	4	5	5	5
Vegetables	2	2	2	3	3	3	3
Complex carbohydrates	7	8	9	9	9	10	11
Protein	2	2	2	2	2	3	3
Fats	2	3	3	3	3	3	3
Dairy and nondairy	2	2	2	2	2	2	2

Suppose you've determined on a personal daily calorie intake of 1430 calories, factoring in your sex, age, and activity level. That puts you in the 1400-calorie column on the chart, and that means that you should eat, every day: four servings of fruit, two servings of vegetables, seven servings of whole grains, two servings of legumes or other protein, two servings of nuts and seeds or oils, and two servings of dairy or nondairy foods.

What constitutes a serving? The pages that follow define what constitutes a serving for basic foods in each of the five PowerFood categories and for dairy and nondairy foods as well. Each portion shown equals one serving. For example, look under complex carbohydrates. Half a bagel constitutes one serving. So at that 1430-calorie-per-day level, calling for seven complex carbohydrate servings a day, half a bagel for breakfast is only one seventh of the desired daily intake. If breakfast included the other half of the bagel (one serving) plus half a cup of oatmeal (one serving) sprinkled with a quarter cup of wheat germ (one serving), that would total four of the desired complex carbohydrate servings; add half a cup of low-fat milk on the cereal, and that equals half of one of the two dairy servings the individual should be having each day. The charts that follow give some indication of the wide-ranging choices available for putting together a personal PowerFoods plan at any level of daily calorie intake—dramatic evidence of the boundless variety in the PowerFoods way of eating.

Fruits

Fruits are Nature's sweet treats, providing quick energy in a delicious, ready-to-eat package. In addition to their phytochemical power, they are an excellent source of vitamins A and C, potassium, and fiber. One serving of fruit is equivalent to about 80 calories.

Vegetables

Vegetables give more nutrient bang for the calorie than any other category of food. They are a rich source of vitamins A, C, E, and K, of minerals, and of fiber, as well as offering abundant phytochemicals. Vegetables are great for snacks, side dishes, salads, and entrées. Raw or cooked, they are superb sources of energy and health. Of course, when

Fruit

1 Serving Equals

Apple	1	*Mango*	1
Applesauce	1 cup	*Nectarines*	2
Apricots	4	*Orange*	1
Apricots, dried	4	*Papaya*	1
Banana	1	*Peaches*	2
Blackberries	2 cups	*Pear, small*	2
Blueberries	1½ cups	*Pears, dried*	2
Cantaloupe	½	*Pineapple*	1 cup
Cherries	20	*Plums*	4
Dates	4	*Prunes, dried*	4
Figs, fresh	2	*Raisins*	4 tablespoons
Figs, dried	2	*Raspberries*	2 cups
Grapefruit	1	*Strawberries*	2 cups
Grapes	15	*Tangerines*	2
Honeydew	½	*Watermelon*	2 cups

it comes to versatility in combining with other foods, vegetables have no peer.

Each serving of vegetables in the following chart is equivalent to about 60 calories. For all the vegetables listed, one cup equals one serving cooked. Uncooked vegetables literally don't count; eat them as often as desired.

Vegetables

1 Serving Equals 1 Cup

Asparagus	*Cabbage—all kinds*
Bean sprouts	*Carrots*
Beets	*Cauliflower*
Broccoli	*Celery*
Brussels sprouts	*Cucumbers*

(continued)

Eggplant	*Mushrooms*
Greens	*Okra*
Beet	*Onions*
Chard	*Radishes*
Chicory	*Rutabaga*
Collard	*Red peppers*
Kale	*String beans*
Lettuce	*Summer squash*
Mustard	*Turnips*
Parsley	*Wax beans*
Spinach	*Zucchini*
Watercress	

Complex Carbohydrates

Complex carbohydrates include starchy vegetables, whole grains, and legumes. They provide the high-energy carbohydrate fuel for your active lifestyle. These foods are rich in B-complex vitamins; in such minerals as iron, calcium, and phosphorous; in both soluble and insoluble fiber; and in phytochemicals. One serving of complex carbohydrates is equivalent to some 70 calories.

All the complex carbohydrates contain some protein. This is particularly the case with the legumes. In counting, therefore, you may consider half a cup of legumes as a serving of either complex carbohydrates or of protein. In general, on days when you are eating animal protein, count legumes as complex carbohydrate. When you are relying on legumes as your sole source of protein, count them as protein. *Do not* count legumes as both complex carbohydrate and protein at the same meal.

Protein

Meat, chicken, and fish are good protein sources, but keep in mind that they are not a good source of fiber. In addition, meat, chicken, and fish must be selected and prepared carefully to ensure that they are as fat-free as possible. A serving of these protein foods is equivalent to 110 calories.

Complex Carbohydrates

	1 Serving Equals
Cooked legumes (dried beans, peas, lentils)	½ cup
Corn on the cob	1
Parsnips	⅔ cup
Potato, white	1 medium
Pumpkin	½ cup
Winter squash	½ cup
Sweet potato or yam	½ medium
Dry cereal, flakes	⅔ cup
Dry cereal, puffed	1½ cups
Grits, cooked	½ cup
Oatmeal and other hot cereals	½ cup
Pasta	½ cup
Popcorn (no fat added)	3 cups
Brown rice, cooked	½ cup
Wheat germ	½ cup
Barley	½ cup
Quinoa	½ cup
Amaranth	½ cup
Bagel	½
Corn bread	1 cube, 2″ × 2″
English muffin	½
Graham crackers	2
Melba toast	4
Pumpernickel	1 slice
Ry-Krisp	3
Rye bread	1 slice
Whole wheat bread	1 slice

Proteins

	1 Serving Equals
Tofu and tempeh	4 ounces
Chicken, turkey, Cornish hen–skinless meat	2 ounces
Any fresh or frozen fish	2 ounces
Canned salmon, tuna, mackerel, crab, lobster	½ cup
Clams, mussels, oysters, scallops, shrimp	10 each
Sardines, drained or water-packed	6 each
Beef: chuck, flank steak, tenderloin, skirt steak, top or bottom round, rump, lean spareribs	2 ounces
Veal: leg, loin, rib, shank, shoulder, cutlets	2 ounces
Lamb: leg, sirloin, rib or loin chops, shank, shoulder	2 ounces
Pork: leg, lean ham, center-cut loin chops	2 ounces
Eggs: poached, boiled, scrambled, omelet	1 extra large

Fats

Nuts, seeds, and oils are high in calories, but they contain essential fatty acids necessary for healthy cell structure. The PowerFood answer to the aren't-they-fattening? question is to eat them in small amounts. Where the oils are concerned, remember that vegetable oils, which are usually liquid at room temperature, are polyunsaturated or monounsaturated, while fats of animal origin, solid at room temperature, are saturated and should be avoided. A serving of nuts, seeds, and oils is equivalent to 45 calories.

Dairy and Nondairy

Dairy products provide protein but contain varying amounts of saturated fat and cholesterol and must be chosen with care. Read the labels; they're your guide to fat content. Then choose fat-free or low-fat items as much as possible. The plus side of dairy products—and of such nondairy products as rice milk and soy cheese—is that they are an excellent source of calcium for strong, healthy bones and teeth. If fortified, these products also contain vitamins A and D. A serving of these foods is equivalent to some 80 calories.

PowerFoods

Fats

	1 Serving Equals
Avocado	⅛
Olives	8 small
Almonds	10
Pecans	2
Walnuts	6
Spanish peanuts	20
Virginia peanuts	10
Polyunsaturated plant oils: *corn, soy, sunflower, safflower*	1 teaspoon
Monounsaturated plant oils: *olive, peanut*	1 teaspoon
Mayonnaise (*made with polyunsaturated oil*)	1 teaspoon
Salad dressing (*made with polyunsaturated oil*)	2 teaspoons
Butter	1 teaspoon
Sour cream, light cream	2 tablespoons

Dairy and Nondairy Products

	1 Serving Equals
Skim milk	1 cup
Powdered milk	⅓ cup
Buttermilk	1 cup
Yogurt, nonfat	1 cup
1 percent milk	1 cup
2 percent milk	½ cup
Cottage cheese (*up to 2 percent fat*)	½ cup
Part-skim milk cheeses: *mozzarella, ricotta, Jarlsberg, Neufchâtel, farmer's*	1½ ounces
Whole-milk cheeses: *Cheddar, Swiss, Muenster, provolone, Gouda, Edam, Parmesan, Romano*	1 ounce

A Plan, Not a Chart

Let's put it all together, using the example of our fifty-year-old woman. She weighs 140 pounds, and she leads an inactive life, but she has decided to change all that. In fact, her doctor has told her that her blood pressure is a bit high, and that her blood sugar and triglyceride levels are increasing. Given the family history of diabetes, she could be heading for trouble if she doesn't lose weight, increase her activity level, change her behavior. She is at the midpoint of her life, and she is resolved that the rest of her life will be lived healthily.

To lose weight, she has modified her age-adjusted BMR to 1593—below the level she would need to maintain her current weight. She is also determined to follow a routine of regular exercise; she has joined a gym and has signed up for an aerobics class three times a week. That means she should raise her intake somewhat—to 1700 calories per day. Her daily food plan would therefore include: four servings of fruit, three servings of vegetables, nine servings of whole grains, two servings of legumes or other proteins, three servings of nuts and seeds or their oils, and two servings of dairy.

But, given what her doctor has discovered about her particular health condition—high triglycerides and high blood sugar—she will do better with a slightly higher level of protein and, believe it or not, of fat: the right kind of fat, as in nuts, seeds, olives, and avocados. So in her case, given her desired daily calorie intake, she might exchange three servings of whole grains for two of protein and one of fat. That would change her daily food plan slightly to include four servings of legumes or other proteins, four servings of nuts and seeds and their oils, and just seven servings of whole grains, as well as four fruit and three vegetable servings.

Simple. What's more, looking at the preceding food charts or glancing at the recipes in Part Four makes it clear that our fifty-year-old has some delicious eating ahead of her, not to mention a healthier life. The same will be true for you.

Your PowerFoods Weight Loss Plan

Keep track. Use the table that follows as your guide. Make copies of this table so that you can keep track day after day. Fill in the number of servings of each food category your food plan provides for you to eat each day, then record the foods you actually did eat that day, measuring them not in calories, or grams, but as pieces of fruit, servings of vegetables, number of nuts. At the end of each day, add up the number of servings actually eaten in each category and compare it to the recommended number. If, for example, you have eaten more fat and less fruit than recommended, make a mental note to have less fat and more fruit tomorrow.

Keep on keeping track until it becomes second nature—and it will—until you can walk past a buffet table making healthy choices, until you just look at a plate of food and know that it's good for you.

My Personal PowerFoods Weight Loss Plan

	Fruits	Vegetables	Complex carbo-hydrates	Proteins	Fats	Dairy and nondairy
# Servings recommended for today						
Breakfast						
Snack						
Lunch						
Snack						
Dinner						
Snack						
# Servings eaten today						

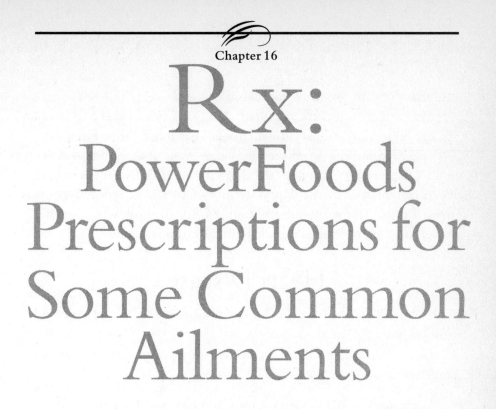

Chapter 16

Rx:
PowerFoods
Prescriptions for
Some Common
Ailments

"Healing,"
Papa would tell me,
"is not a science,
but the intuitive art
of wooing Nature."
—W. H. AUDEN

*t*he times we live in seem to breed
a particular brand of diseases and conditions, as our bodies try to cope
with the stresses and strains of modern industrial societies and with
the toxic pollutants introduced into our environment in the twentieth
century. What's more, many of our era's afflictions are chronic and
degenerative in nature. Of course, the century has also produced stun-
ning advances in medical knowledge and medical treatments.
Increasingly, however, the findings of medical research encourage the
prevention of these diseases, and they support my firmly held convic-

tion that the path to prevention lies in changes in diet and behavior.

My patients often ask me what changes they can make to guard against these ailments. My short answer? Eat more PowerFoods and less of everything else. (And keep moving—more about physical activity in Chapter 18.) Of course, the short answer isn't always enough, so when patients ask what I would do myself, or what I would recommend for my husband and children, I offer the following specific PowerFoods prescriptions for what ails far too many of us.

Heart Disease

Let's start with the nation's number one killer of men and women: heart disease.

First, concentrate on PowerFoods with a proven ability to lower cholesterol:

○ **Soy protein—Eat soybeans, tofu, tempeh, soy burgers, soy milk, soy cheese, soy yogurt, soy nuts, and soy flour. "Skimmed" versions of soy foods contain less fat than "regular" soy foods; these are increasingly available in markets everywhere.**
○ **Garlic and company—Add some flavor to your meals with garlic, onions, shallots, leeks, scallions, and chives; all these members of the allium family deliver natural cholesterol protection.**

Second, rev up your intake of PowerFoods with proven antioxidant abilities. Oxidation of LDL, the "bad" cholesterol, is thought to be one of the first steps in clogging blood vessels with fatty plaque. A diet focusing on PowerFoods rich in antioxidants strengthens your defense against cholesterol buildup:

○ **Carrots, sweet potatoes, yams, pumpkins, squash, kale, broccoli, cantaloupe—all great sources of the powerful carotenoid antioxidants**
○ **Cucumber—a source of cholesterol-lowering sterols**
○ **Citrus fruits—provide terpenes to decrease arterial plaque.**

Third, bump up fiber. Soluble fibers act like a cholesterol sponge and aid in clearing LDL cholesterol from your body. Insoluble fibers aid in elimination. Aim to consume at least 25 grams of fiber per day:

○ **Legumes (beans, peas, and lentils), oatmeal and oat bran, barley, fruits, and vegetables are high in soluble fiber.**

○ **Whole grains such as wheat and rye, wheat bran, and rice bran are high in the insoluble fibers.**

Fourth, take the low-fat route, but make sure that you consume at least fifteen grams of fat per day—less than that can lower the HDL or "good" cholesterol. Remember that our goal is to increase HDL while lowering LDL. Fifteen grams of fat per day amounts to very, very little fat. For number lovers, here's the math:

Fat has nine calories per gram. Fifteen grams therefore contains 135 calories (15×9). That would be only 10 percent of the total calories required by an individual on a 1350-calorie-per-day diet ($1350 \times 10\% = 135$). For food plans of 1400 to 2000 calories, 15 grams of fat would be less than 10 percent in all cases. There's an important lesson here: no more fear of fat. Just look at the following table to see how many grams of fat constitute the required 10 to 20 percent you should be eating at your particular daily calorie level.

Recommended Fat Intake Guide

Calories Per Day	Fat Grams As Percentage of Daily Intake	
	10%	20%
1400	16	32
1500	17	34
1600	18	36
1700	19	38
1800	20	40
1900	21	42
2000	22	44

Of course, you should choose fats wisely. Minimize saturated and hydrogenated fats. The saturated fats are found primarily in such animal foods as meats and poultry, and in the dairy products milk, cheese, and butter. Hydrogenated fats are artificially created by changing a liquid vegetable oil into a solid form. The end result of the process is unhealthy in two ways: it raises the "bad" LDL and lowers the "good" HDL. That makes hydrogenated fats completely counterproductive, so when you see the words "partially hydrogenated" on the label of such processed foods as margarine, baked goods, coffee creamers, snack foods, and candy, avoid them.

Instead, the following PowerFoods provide the healthy monounsaturated fats:

○ **Olives and avocados—the high-fat vegetables**
○ **Nuts and seeds—especially walnuts, almonds, flax seeds, sesame, pumpkin and sunflower seeds**
○ **Oils from vegetables, nuts, and seeds—canola, flax seed, olive, peanut, sesame, and walnut oils. Remember to use these in moderation. One teaspoon of oil provides 5 grams of fat.**

A word about lowering triglyceride levels. High triglyceride levels are often found in people with excess weight around the middle of their body—the so-called "apple" shape. Often there is a family history of noninsulin-dependent diabetes (NIDDM, also called Type II diabetes). Frequently, the HDL cholesterol levels are low as well. Weight loss is usually the first step; get that waist size back to what it was before the extra pounds arrived. The ideal food plan includes the monounsaturated fats with a total fat intake that is about 20 percent of daily calories; it also minimizes processed grain products like pasta, bagels, pretzels, and crackers. Lean meat and poultry can be eaten in moderation.

To add variety to your healthy-heart PowerFoods plan, enjoy fish and shellfish several times a week. Fish oil contains omega–3 fatty acids, which have been shown to lower triglyceride levels, increase HDL levels, prevent blood clots, and improve blood pressure. Fatty fish—tuna, salmon, bluefish, mackerel, herring, and sardines—are the best source of omega 3. Shellfish are very low in saturated fat, so enjoy shrimp, lobster, mussels, clams, and scallops, but hold the butter, cream sauce, and rich stuffing. Boiled, broiled, steamed, and stir-fried are the preferred cooking methods.

Hypertension

Closely associated with heart disease is hypertension—high blood pressure—a common condition affecting 60 million adults in the United States. What is particularly scary about hypertension is that it is usually symptom-free and is therefore often undiagnosed. It is thus a stealthy killer—a major risk factor for both heart disease and stroke.

Physicians and patients typically turn to medication to lower blood pressure. While medication often works, it has the potential to cause side effects. Besides, the quick fix promise of drugs overlooks the often profound benefits available from changes in lifestyle. Such changes—in nutrition, level of physical activity, and relaxation—have proven to be highly effective, and their only side effect is to improve all aspects of the individual's health.

The most effective lifestyle change for anyone suffering hypertension, or worried about suffering it, is weight loss. Even a small loss of weight can have a significant effect. Over the long term, translate that life-style change into eating more PowerFoods and less of everything else—and remaining physically active. That is the secret of success for permanent weight loss.

PowerFoods that may work specifically to lower blood pressure are typically high in potassium and magnesium and include:

○ **Fruits—apricots, bananas, berries, grapefruit, grapes, mangoes, melons, nectarines, oranges, and peaches**
○ **Legumes—chick-peas, kidney beans, pinto beans, lentils, peas, and soybeans in all forms**
○ **Vegetables—artichokes, broccoli, carrots, cauliflower, potatoes, spinach.**

Osteoporosis

Osteoporosis is that condition of "porous bones" that particularly—but not exclusively—affects older women. The decrease in bone mass and bone density typically leads to painful and disabling fractures and causes the signature "dowager's hump" often visible on stooped elderly women. Osteoporosis affects one out of every four postmenopausal women in the United States, causing approximately 1.3 million fractures a year. Because almost a quarter of women who fracture a hip will die in the year following the fracture, osteoporosis is clearly far more than a disfiguring ache.

The major risk factor for osteoporosis is a chronic shortage of calcium. It is estimated that American women are taking in half—or less than half—of the recommended daily amount (RDA) of calcium in their diets. In fact, recent research suggests that 1200 to 1500 milligrams of calcium per day is required. What's more, adequate vitamin D is needed in order for the body to absorb and use the calcium properly.

Dairy foods are an obvious way to ensure calcium intake, but they are by no means the only way. A number of other foods also provide calcium—the leafy green PowerFoods, tofu, blackstrap molasses, the soft bones in canned sardines and salmon, beans and whole grains, figs, apricots, and rhubarb. As for vitamin D, it is found in fortified milk and in a limited number of foods, and it is made by the body when skin is exposed to sunlight. (Fifteen minutes of sunlight twice a week ought to do it for young adults; for the elderly, more than that is recommended.)

Here are some foods that are particularly good sources of calcium:

○ **Dried beans**
○ **Whole grains**
○ **Dark green leafy vegetables (broccoli, bok choy, mustard, collard, turnip greens, kale, and others)**
○ **Figs**
○ **Apricots**
○ **Rhubarb**

- ○ Calcium-fortified orange juice
- ○ Yogurt, nonfat or low-fat
- ○ Milk, skim or low-fat
- ○ Nonfat dry milk powder
- ○ Calcium-fortified soy milk
- ○ Sardines with bones
- ○ Canned salmon with bones
- ○ Tofu
- ○ Blackstrap molasses

In addition to diet, exercise is essential—especially weight-bearing exercise and strength training.

Cancer

Cancer is perhaps the most dreaded scourge of our age. While it is no longer the automatic "death sentence" it once was, thanks to outstanding advances in therapy and treatment, it still kills more than 500,000 Americans annually.

Perhaps the best and simplest protection against cancer is the low-fat, high-fiber way of eating that is the basic PowerFoods plan. In addition to the red, yellow, and orange fruits and vegetables loaded with cancer-preventing, antioxidant carotenoids, the cruciferous vegetables must be a particular focus: broccoli, bok choy, brussels sprouts, green or red cabbage, cauliflower, rutabaga, turnips, kale, collards, and the greens of mustard, beet, and turnip. And remember garlic and company, mushrooms, nuts and seeds, legumes, whole grains, and sea vegetables.

This entire book is a cancer prevention prescription. Carefully read each of the chapters on the individual PowerFoods groups to learn how certain foods have the power to prevent certain cancers.

Chapter 17

You Can Choose Your Actions— The Results Are a Gift

You must not expect anything from others. It's you yourself of whom you must ask a lot. Only from oneself has one the right to ask everything or anything. This way it's up to you—your choice. What you get from others remains a present, a gift.
—ALBERT SCHWEITZER

*N*ow that you have a food plan, of course, you must follow it. No one else can do that for you. By the same token, what, how, and when you eat are entirely within your control. After all, it is your hand reaching out for the food, your mouth taking it in, your voice saying either "Yes, please" or "No, thank you" to your host's offer of a second or third helping. You control your food choices, portion sizes, and whether or not you eat regularly through-out the day or, as one of my patients put it, "like a dog," wolfing down one large, frenzied meal each evening without much notice of what you're eating and with less appreciation. Following your food plan is within your control—and it is your choice.

Of course, in undertaking any plan, it's important to have a goal in mind. But there is a certain kind of goal-setting that is simply an invi-tation to failure. Suppose you decide you want to lose twenty pounds in the next three months in order to make an impression at your son's wedding, or your daughter's graduation, or your twenty-fifth reunion. What if you only lose ten pounds? You feel you've failed. Once again, you have disappointed yourself; the result is unhappiness.

Now suppose instead that you choose to focus on *actions,* on eat-ing more PowerFoods and less of everything else—without a time frame or a specified number of pounds. At the end of three months, you receive a gift of a ten-pound weight loss and a bonus of enhanced energy, smooth skin, and shiny hair. Instead of the disappointment you felt because you failed to lose twenty pounds, you now feel pleased with your new sense of control. You feel confident in your lifetime food plan, certain that you will lose the weight you want to lose—permanently. So focus on your actions, not on specific results, and it will follow, as day follows night, that the desired results will come, in their own way and in their own time.

But let's say that after three months, you have lost only a few pounds, and you're not feeling any particular bonus burst of well-being. Don't get mad, and don't give up. Again, focus on your actions: Are you eating more PowerFoods but also more of everything else? Are you still pretty much a couch potato? Change your actions—food choices, portion size. Get up and get moving. (More about that in the next chapter.) Keep your goal on changing the process, and the results must change in due course.

Psychologists tell us that it takes 22 tries to form a habit. So if you're trying to counter an old habit of snacking on potato chips with a new snack of fruit, three fruits a day for a week could conceivably create a healthy habit that lasts a lifetime. Similarly, working out to a video every Monday, Wednesday and Friday morning could become routine in 2 months. Be sure to recognize such actions for the successes they are; when you counter bad behavior with good, applaud yourself. The reward will be the gift of good health.

Power Pointers

Here are some pointers for practical problem-solving as you go about changing your behavior and following your personal PowerFoods Plan.

Shopping Pointers

Shop in the outside aisles of your grocery store or supermarket. Fresh foods—fruits and vegetables, bins of whole grains and legumes and nuts and seeds, fresh meat, fish, and poultry, fresh dairy products—are typically sold around the perimeter of the store. They surround the inner aisles filled with processed foods in boxes, cans, or plastic containers. These processed foods are typically higher in fat and salt and should be avoided.

If you must buy prepackaged food, read the label. Compare similar items and choose the one with the lowest fat content. This is especially easy to do in the dairy department, where skim milk and low-fat cheese and yogurt are clearly marked and prominently displayed.

Don't buy products made with ingredients that are high in saturated fats and cholesterol: butter, lard, hydrogenated vegetable oil, coconut and palm oil, cream or cream sauces, whole milk solids, and cheese.

PowerFood Recipe Repair

Question the need for each individual ingredient. For high-fat or high-cholesterol ingredients, decide if they can be eliminated, substituted, or at least reduced. For example, you can reduce the amount of fat and cholesterol in soups, stews, and casseroles and increase your consumption of PowerFoods by substituting beans and grains for meat.

Compile a list of "insteads." Be creative. Instead of a juicy steak, try a juicy portobello mushroom, grilled and seasoned the same way as you would the steak. Here are some more replacement suggestions:

Instead of:	Use:
whole milk	skim milk, soy milk, rice milk
cream	evaporated skim milk
butter or lard	olive, flax seed, or walnut oil
sour cream or mayonnaise	low-fat yogurt, low-fat soy yogurt
high-fat cheese	part-skim cheese, part-skim soy cheese
meat, chicken, fish	beans, peas, lentils, whole grains.

In addition to ingredient replacement, be creative with cooking methods. Instead of fried potatoes, try baking potato wedges seasoned with a blend of herbs and with a touch of Parmesan cheese. Thin sauces or soups by adding fruit or vegetable juice; thicken soups and stews with starchy vegetables. Create new kinds of toppings. Instead of sour cream, use ricotta cheese or yogurt cheese, add herbs, finely chopped vegetables, and perhaps a dash of Tabasco. The result makes a new kind of sandwich spread as well as a potato topping. Or, mix yogurt cheese or nonfat cream cheese with cinnamon, vanilla, and chopped fresh or dried fruit for a sweet topping on cereals, pancakes, toast—or on its own for a dessert.

Try new combinations:

○ **exotic vegetables like kohlrabi, jicama, daikon, radicchio, fennel tossed with such greens as endive, escarole, romaine, spinach**

○ **salads of carrots and apples, oranges and sweet potatoes, pumpkin and pears**

○ **shredded carrots, diced peppers, sliced radishes, chopped olives, green onion, chopped tomato, sliced cucumber mixed with nonfat cottage cheese.**

Think new thoughts. Try a blended fruit, yogurt, and cinnamon shake for breakfast or lunch. Designate a weekly clean-out-the-fridge night, when all leftover vegetables are thrown into a soup pot to which you add any other spare ingredients and some unusual seasonings. Or experiment with a different whole grain per week until you've gone from amaranth to quinoa, stopping at barley, kasha, and millet along the way.

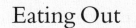

Eating Out

You can and should follow your food plan no matter where you eat, even in restaurants. Start by assessing your hunger level before going out to eat. If you're moderately hungry, you can look forward to being in control of ordering a good meal that follows your personal food plan. If you're very hungry, have a low-calorie snack before leaving home. I call that "preventive eating."

Once you confront the menu, stay in control to make the right choices, and be prepared to articulate special requests with your waiter. Keep in mind that the restaurant's management wants to please you, the customer, and will be willing to make menu modifications to a reasonable extent.

If you order an appetizer, stick to clear soup, raw vegetables, fresh fruit cocktail, and tomato juice; avoid such items as cream soups, fried tidbits, and cheese dips. When the bread basket is passed around, avoid white bread and crackers, but if you see whole grain bread or rolls, enjoy either one slice or just one roll, without butter. Ask to have your vegetables steamed and served without butter or cheese sauce. Don't add butter or sour cream to that baked potato. If you can't get the vegetables you want the way you want them prepared, have an extra large salad instead. Ask for the dressing on the side and use it sparingly—no more than one tablespoon. Lemon juice or vinegar alone will make delicious alternatives, and they're calorie-free; any restaurant should accommodate you if you ask for them.

Ask if there are any vegetarian specials—for example, vegetarian chili or a vegetable stir-fry. If you order chicken or fish, no cream sauce, butter, or gravy. Instead, ask for seasonings made with herbs, spices, dry white wine, lemon juice, mushrooms, tomatoes, green pepper, onions, and garlic. Broiling, steaming, and baking are the cooking methods of choice.

As for dessert, think fruit. Better yet, before ordering any dessert, stop and ask yourself if you're still hungry. If the answer is no, just stop. You might like that piece of fruit a little later at home.

Count Your Blessings

Finally, count your blessings, *not* calories, grams of fat, numbers of vitamins, even phytochemical content. Nature has provided a glorious bounty of health-giving, life-enhancing foods. We have access to all of it—as close as your kitchen garden in many cases, but certainly no farther than the nearest supermarket.

The recipes in Part Four fit every food plan; they're easy to make and guaranteed to provide PowerFoods for all occasions and all circumstances. Make them your starting point for your PowerFoods program. There's no need to count calories, grams, or anything else with these recipes. Of course, you might want to exercise some caution when it comes to the Apricot Bread Pudding in Chapter 27: just one serving please, and just once in a while. But remember: In a lifetime eating plan, it's okay to splurge when the occasion calls for it.

The food we have available to us is really a blessing—a generous gift to nourish and nurture. So as you change your behavior to eat more PowerFoods and less of everything else, be grateful.

Chapter 18

Keep Moving

I wish to preach, not the doctrine of ignoble ease, but the doctrine of the strenuous life.

—THEODORE ROOSEVELT

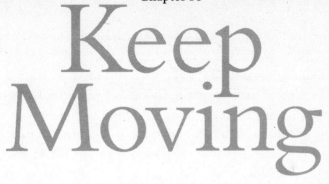

*i*f the PowerFoods program puts PowerFoods first in your way of eating, it puts exercise first in your way of living. The value of physical exercise is so well established as to be unarguable. Study after study after study proclaims the need for exercise by the very old as well as the very young, by the disabled as well as athletes, by those who work in factories or offices as well as those who farm the fields or drive trucks or dig ditches or patrol our national parks for a living.

Recent research powerfully and dramatically demonstrates that regular exercise can actually counteract destructive health habits; that it can in many cases (but only up to a certain point) compensate for unhealthy eating; that it helps people react positively to work pressures; and that vigorous exercise can actually prolong life by increasing circulation enough to strengthen the heart.

Certainly, physically fit people are not entirely immune from illness, injury, the debilitating effects of aging. But for the most part, their illnesses are more easily borne, they recover more quickly from their injuries, and they age later and with less impact than the unfit. People who are physically active tend to live longer, and while they live, they feel better because of the exercise they get.

Exercise isn't just beneficial, it's essential, and no PowerFoods program is complete without a fitness program of regular exercise. There are many definitions of fitness, to be sure, and there are as many styles of fitness "workout" as there are individuals. Most experts now agree that a comprehensive exercise program should include—with regular, alternating repetition—aerobic activity for cardiovascular fitness, weight-bearing exercise and resistance training for strength, and stretching for flexibility.

Cardiovascular exercise improves the ability of the heart and blood vessels to supply oxygen to your body so that vital organs perform at peak efficiency. Cardiovascular fitness is essential to body maintenance, growth, and repair; the more oxygen supplied and used, the greater the body's total work capacity.

Weight-bearing exercise builds strong bones; it's a good preventive measure against osteoporosis and bone fractures later in life. While many of the aerobic activities essential to cardiovascular health are weight-bearing—walking, jogging, hiking, climbing stairs—some are not. Swimming, cycling, and rowing, all marvelously healthful activities, are not specifically weight-bearing. Resistance training, which includes weight-lifting and working out on those resistance machines in the local gym or health club, builds and tones muscles. Since the body tends to lose muscle mass with age, resistance training can help keep your muscles fit and flexible as you grow older. Although it's a cliché to say that if you don't use it, you lose it, it is a medical fact.

Hand in hand with strength training is flexibility training—stretching for warm-up and cool-down. Stretching reduces the internal resistance offered by soft connective tissues; this loosens and elongates the tissue, thus lessening the likelihood of injury. It is not known exactly how this works, but most researchers suspect that stretching stimulates the production or retention of lubricants between the connective tissue fibers, thus preventing the formation of adhesions. Whatever the precise reason, it is certain that without stretching, the connective tissue will begin to fray and lose elasticity, and the muscles will stiffen and lose flexibility. Aging has some of the same effects on connective tissue, so stretching throughout a lifetime is an excellent idea.

Of course, before you begin any exercise program, check with your doctor.

Your Personal Exercise Prescription

The United States in the last years of the twentieth century offers an abundance—almost an excess—of exercise options. Just check the yellow pages, monitor the ads in your newspaper, or browse the World Wide Web to scratch the surface of the possibilities. Spas, gyms, exercise equipment, activity vacations abound. You can choose step classes, racquetball, a personal trainer, t'ai chi, a home ski machine, a vigorous mountain bike ride, a brisk walk in the park at lunchtime. Or all of the above, alternating a different exercise on different days so that you don't become bored. What you choose as your exercise doesn't matter; what counts is that the exercise be rhythmic and continuous—keep moving.

Of course, different types of activity burn different numbers of calories. The more strenuous the activity, the more calories are burned; that means you must take in more calories to meet your daily requirement. An hour's workout on the resistance-machine circuit at your gym could warrant adding as much as 30 percent of your age-adjusted BMR to your desired daily calorie intake. A day of cross-country skiing could more than double your desired daily calorie intake. A morning spent cleaning house, followed by an afternoon of driving the kids to their various appointments, however, will make a barely noticeable difference in desired calorie intake; you'll still need real exercise. The table that follows shows you how much energy is expended in various activities. Obviously, many of these activities combine cardiovascular, weight-bearing, and resistance-training benefits.

In creating your personal prescription for exercise, four factors should be considered, whatever type of exercise you choose: frequency, duration, intensity, and warm-up and cool-down.

The Energy You Use,
The Calories You Burn

Activity	Calories per hour
Light Activity	50–200
Lying down or sleeping	80
Sitting	100
Driving an automobile	120
Standing	140
House cleaning	180
Yoga	200
Moderate Activity	200–350
Bicycling (5 ½ mph), walking (2 ½ mph)	210
Gardening	220
Canoeing (2 ½ mph)	230
Judo, karate, calisthenics	250
Golf	250
Lawn mowing (power mower)	250
Lawn mowing (hand mower)	270
Bowling	270
Baseball, softball	300
Swimming (¼ mph)	300
Walking (3 ¾ mph)	300
Horseback riding (trotting)	350
Square dancing	350
Weight lifting	350
Roller-skating	350
Basketball, football, soccer, volleyball	350
Vigorous Activity	over 350
Ditch digging, snow shoveling, wood chopping	400
Ice skating (10 mph)	400
Tennis (singles)	420

Water skiing	480
Back-packing, hiking	490
Rowing machine	600
Skiing (downhill 10 mph)	600
Jogging (10 min/mile)	600
Squash, handball, racquetball	600
Bicycling (13 mph)	650
Running (7.5 min/mile)	800
Rope jumping	800
Stair climbing	900
Running (6 min/mile)	900
Skiing (cross-country)	1200

Frequency

Basically, you need three or four exercise sessions per week. It's the recurring nature of the activity—the continuity—that achieves optimal cardiovascular functioning, maintains bone strength, and enhances muscle health over time. Sporadic bursts of exercise are as fruitless for the body's conditioning as intermittent crash dieting is for a trim weight and nutritious eating.

But that needn't mean exercising every day. Quite the opposite. Muscles become frayed and need time to repair themselves—more time the older we get; that's why exercising every other day is a good idea. Very often, people just starting an exercise program will be driven by a gung-ho attitude to go all-out, but too much exercise when you're not in condition can be both a turnoff and actually dangerous. So ease into your exercise program, and, especially at the start, give your body time to recover.

Intensity

Intensity—that is, the level of exercise activity—is an absolutely individual matter. Everybody has his or her exercise target zone, corresponding to approximately 60 to 75 percent of the person's maximum work capacity. Very fit, healthy people can exercise at a slightly higher target zone of 65 to 85 percent. Your target zone is expressed as a range of heart rates within which you can exercise safely and beneficially. Once you have computed your target zone, you can monitor your pulse during your exercise session. If you're below your zone, increase the intensity of your exercise; if you're above your zone, slow your pace to decrease your intensity. Here's how to compute your target heart rate zone:

Step 1: Subtract your age from 220 to estimate your maximal heart rate

Step 2: Multiply your maximal heart rate by 60 percent (Line 1 × .60)

Step 3: Multiply your maximal heart rate by 75 percent (Line 1 × .75)

Your target exercise zone is the range between these two numbers. It is often easier while exercising to use a 10-second pulse count. To get the number of beats per 10 seconds, divide each of the target-zone numbers by 6.

Take the example of our fifty-year-old woman. Subtracting her age from 220 yields the number 170. She multiplies 170 by 60 percent to get 102; she multiplies 170 by 75 percent to get 128. Her target heart rate is 102 to 128 pulse beats per minute, or 17 to 23 beats per 10 seconds.

Of course, a changed set of conditions may require you to change your intensity level. During a heat wave, you would have to decrease intensity to stay within your target zone. Improved conditioning is another change that can affect intensity. The more you exercise, the more efficient your body becomes, forcing you to increase the intensity of your exercise activity to maintain your target zone rate.

Duration

Intermittent bursts of feverish exercise separated by restful chats at the health club water cooler not only do you little good, the practice can actually be harmful. What you want is thirty minutes of sustained activity within your target zone. Work up to it. Start with ten minutes of continuous exercise for a week or two, and build up gradually to twenty minutes and then thirty. Exhausting yourself and your body by going all out too soon will just force you back to square one.

Warm-up and Cool-down

Warm-up and cool-down are important for preventing injury and for ensuring a safe, comfortable exercise session. Slow, smooth stretching exercises prepare the muscles and joints and safely start the move from resting pulse rate up toward the target zone. After a few minutes of gentle stretching, ease into the exercise activity itself—jogging, rowing, racquetball—at a modest pace and a low-energy level. After ten minutes of warm-up, you should be at the lower limit of your target zone—ready for thirty minutes of a workout.

When the thirty-minute workout is over, cool-down returns the body to resting pulse rate safely and comfortably. It's the exact reverse of the warm-up: Lessen the pace and intensity of your target zone activity, slowing down gradually; then walk around for a few minutes and do some stretching. You're ready for the shower, and for a delicious PowerFoods snack.

A Final Word

These, then, are the essential components of the PowerFoods Program:

○ **Create a food plan, not a diet, and if weight loss is your goal, lose those pounds slowly in order to lose them permanently**

○ **Identify and change inappropriate eating behavior; build the habit of choosing nutrient-rich PowerFoods**

○ **Get moving: exercise regularly and maintain an active lifestyle**

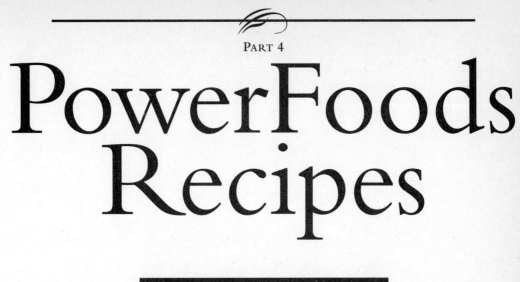

PART 4

PowerFoods
Recipes

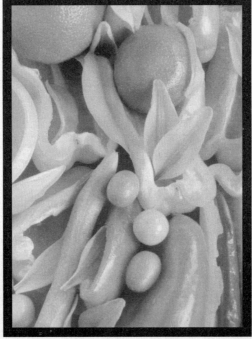

Chapter 19

Putting PowerFoods First

A WAY OF COOKING FOR THE TWENTY-FIRST CENTURY

*t*he PowerFoods principle—putting PowerFoods first in the diet and in menu planning—has afforded me and the chefs at Canyon Ranch in the Berkshires wonderful opportunities to use our creativity. The recipes that follow demonstrate the variety, moderation, and balance available from PowerFoods, the range of tastes possible, and of course, the powerful health benefits a PowerFoods diet provides.

What you won't see here are numbers of calories, cholesterol counts, measures of fat grams, or milligrams of sodium. For one thing, it is no fun to cook by the numbers—no fun for us, and no fun for you. And it is certainly no pleasure to eat by the numbers. Above all, we know that by eating according to the PowerFoods principle, you are getting a diet that is naturally low in calories, fat, and sodium, and that contains low cholesterol (cholesterol is found only in foods of animal origin). That is why the PowerFoods content of each recipe is highlighted. The occasional pat of butter in these recipes, the use of fish or chicken, provides such minimal amounts of fat or cholesterol as to be almost insignificant, while at the same time adding to the taste and texture and sheer pleasure of eating that we believe is so important to a healthy diet. We hope the recipes will serve as a starting point for your own cooking creativity and for the joy of tasty and healthy eating.

Although this book is about the power of phytochemicals in foods, the recipes that follow don't measure phytochemical content any more than they count calories, fat, cholesterol, or sodium. That's because the number of flavonoids in a food, or its concentration of indoles, or the fact that it contains an infection-fighting organosulfur is not reason enough to eat the food.

I began this book by emphasizing that eating is more than just ingesting food in order to live. Eating should be a pleasure, and food should appeal to our senses of vision, smell, and taste as well as answering the cravings of our stomachs. That is why balance, variety, and moderation are the essence of healthy eating; they help you want to eat the foods that are good for you.

William Castelli, the eminent cardiologist and medical researcher who directs the Framingham Heart Study, has said that we could eliminate heart disease from the vast majority of the American public "if everyone would simply adopt ten new healthy recipes."

Begin eating from the 140 PowerFood recipes that follow, and you will be taking a giant step towards a healthier life—for the rest of your life.

Appetizers

Baked Papaya Skewers with Curry Sauce
Sweet Potato Chips
Roasted Peppers
Spinach Hummus
Stuffed Mushrooms

Soups

Carrot Soup
Kale Soup
Cream of Mushroom Soup
Navy Bean Soup
Barbecue Bean Soup
Minestrone

PowerFoods

Borscht
Cinnamon Pumpkin Bisque
Cold Blueberry Soup
Cold Pineapple and Mint Soup

Salads

Apple Coleslaw
Citrus Asparagus Salad
Arugula, Radicchio, and Endive Salad
Arugula and Radicchio Salad with Sherry Vinaigrette
Caesar Salad
Napa Cabbage and Mushroom Salad
Cucumber Salad
Warm Cucumber Salad
Fennel and Cauliflower Salad
Fresh Tomatoes with Mozzarella
Mango and Watercress Salad with Marinated Chicken
Fruited Couscous Salad
Lemon-zested Couscous Dinner Salad
Buckwheat Salad
Brown Rice Salad
Greek Tabbouleh Salad
Hijiki Tossed Salad
Udon and Vegetable Salad
Four-Bean Salad

Vegetable Side Dishes

Beets with Tarragon
Harvard Beets
Sweet and Spiced Baby Carrots
Summer Squash Stir-Fry with Tomatoes
Pattypan Squash Creole
Spaghetti Squash with Pine Nuts
Citrus Butternut Squash
Maple-baked Winter Squash
Honeyed Sweet Potatoes
Sweet-and-Sour Red Cabbage

Turnip Purée
Roasted Red Peppers and Brussels Sprouts
Bok Choy Stir-Fry
Braised Swiss Chard
Steamed Cauliflower with Chive Butter
Stir-fried Broccoli
Creamy Broccoli Casserole
Spinach and Mushroom Stir-Fry
Sweet-and-Sour Onions
Burgundy Mushrooms and Onions
Sautéed Porcini Mushrooms
Lentils with Nori
Dulse Stir-Fry
Marinated Wakame and Zucchini Sticks
Wakame with Parsnips and Carrots
Potatoes with Vegetable Salsa
Southern Succotash
Stuffed Tomatoes with Rice and Pecans
Brown Rice with Burdock
Buckwheat Noodles with Spicy Peanut Sauce
Walnut Bulgur

Entrées
Basil Couscous with Squash
Barley Risotto
Brown Rice Pilaf
Bulgar, Kale, and Carrot Pilaf
Lentil and Brown Rice Casserole
Asian Noodle Salad
Pasta with Papaya Salsa
Pasta with Quick Black Bean Sauce
Pasta with Zucchini Sauce
Root Vegetables and Lamb Stew
Scrambled Tofu Fiesta
Vegetable Chili
Vegetable Calzone

Baked Halibut with Herb Bread Crumb Topping
Baked Trout with Corn Salsa
Grilled Salmon with Fruit Sauce
Salmon Teriyaki
Grilled Tuna Steaks with Ginger Mayonnaise

Sauces, Dressings, and Accompaniments

Tomatillo Salsa
Peanut Saté Dip
Warm Roquefort Dip
Cranberry Chutney
Pineapple Apricot Chutney
Mandarin Poppy Seed Dressing
Miso Vinaigrette
Papaya Vinaigrette
Pineapple Mango Dressing
Tofu Dill Mayonnaise
Barbecue Sauce
Fresh Tomato Sauce
Mushroom Marinara Sauce
Mustard Chive Pasta Sauce
Yellow Pepper Sauce
Pesto
Blueberry Syrup
Orange Cherry Jubilee Sauce
Raspberry Sauce
Peach Butter

Breads, Muffins, and Pancakes

Barry Bread
Corn Bread
Sweet Potato Gingerbread
Pumpkin Bread
Banana Cherry Nut Bread
Bran Muffins
Buckwheat Muffins

Grape-Nuts Muffins
Sweet Potato Muffins
Orange and Fig Muffins
Sweet Potato Pancakes
Rice Flour Pancakes

Desserts
Apple Butter Cake
Apple Cranberry Crisp
Apple Nut Cake
Baked Apples with Cherries and Walnuts
Danish Applesauce
Apricot Blackberry Cobbler
Apricot Poppy Seed Cake
Baked Quince
Fresh Strawberries Chantilly
Gingered Tangerines with Mint
Dried Fruit Turnover
Tropical Fruit Cup
Fruit Compote
Fresh Melon Compote
Cantaloupe Sorbet
Peach Frisée
Pineapple Banana Shake
Blackberry Kanten
Wild Blueberry Loaf
Apricot Raisin Bread Pudding
Basmati Rice Pudding
Papaya Fig Bruschetta
Whole Wheat Crêpes with Blueberry Filling
Tofu Brownies
Chocolate Fondue Dip

Chapter 20

Appetizers

*i*nstead of the usual chips with dips and salted peanuts, offer these healthful, beautiful dishes to whet the appetites of guests. They will satisfy eyes, taste buds, and appetites in a most healthy way. What's more, all these dishes can serve as more than party hors d'oeuvres or meal openers. Consider making them parts of your meals—as side dishes or main dishes.

Baked Papaya Skewers
with Curry Sauce

Serves 6

a break from traditional kabobs, these can be made ahead and then baked or grilled. The pineapple juice and curry enhance the natural sweetness of the papaya, which when baked leaves a melt-in-your-mouth feeling.

2 papayas, peeled and seeded
¼ cup regular or nonfat mayonnaise
1 tablespoon minced fresh chives
1 teaspoon curry powder
¼ teaspoon salt
2 tablespoons pineapple juice
¼ teaspoon freshly ground black pepper
1 dozen 4-inch wooden skewers, soaked in water
    for 30 minutes

1. Preheat the oven to 350°F.
2. Cut the peeled and seeded papayas into ½-inch-thick cubes.
3. In a large, shallow bowl, combine mayonnaise, chives, curry powder, salt, pineapple juice, and black pepper.
4. Thread 3 or 4 papaya cubes on each skewer and place in the sauce. Marinate 30 minutes, turning occasionally. Remove from marinade.
5. Bake on a cookie sheet for 10 to 15 minutes or grill on an outdoor barbecue until the papaya cubes are lightly browned. Serve warm.

POWERFOOD HIGHLIGHT
Papaya, chives, curry powder, pineapple juice

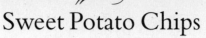

Sweet Potato Chips
Serves 8

*t*hese baked treats are better than any chip that comes in a package—not to mention the hefty dose of carotenoids they offer. Regular potato chips will taste very bland when compared to this tasty chip that needs no dip to accompany it.

4 sweet potatoes
Nonstick vegetable spray

1. Wash the sweet potatoes and cut them very thin, either with a mandoline or very carefully with a sharp knife.
2. Preheat the oven to 400°F.
3. Lightly spray a cookie sheet with vegetable spray coating.
4. Spread the sweet potato slices on the cookie sheet in one layer and spray their tops lightly with vegetable spray. This may take one or two batches, depending on the size of the cookie sheet.
5. Bake until the chips begin to brown, approximately 15 to 20 minutes.

POWERFOOD HIGHLIGHT
Sweet potatoes

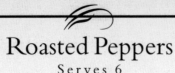

Roasted Peppers
Serves 6

*t*here's nothing like the tempting aroma of a pepper roasting to awaken your taste buds. Smother these over pasta, sandwich them on crusty bread or just savor all alone with a drizzle of olive oil.

2 red bell peppers
2 yellow bell peppers
3 tablespoons freshly squeezed lime juice
¼ teaspoon salt
1 clove garlic, peeled and minced
12 medium pitted black olives, thinly sliced

1. Preheat the broiler. Place the peppers under the broiler until their skins become charred, turning them to ensure that all sides are exposed to the heat. Remove the peppers from the oven and place them in a paper bag.

2. In a mixing bowl combine the lime juice, salt, and garlic. Add the olive slices.

3. Remove the peppers from the bag. Skin and seed them and cut them, lengthwise, into strips.

4. Add the pepper strips to the olive and lime juice mixture. Toss to coat the peppers and then place in the refrigerator. Let stand 1 hour. Serve cool or at room temperature.

POWERFOOD HIGHLIGHT
Peppers, lime juice, garlic, olives

Spinach Hummus
Serves 5

a wonderful departure from the ordinary, this hummus takes minutes to make and presents itself beautifully in a clear glass bowl. Dip it with pita wedges, sesame crackers, or raw veggie slices. This veggie bean dip is perfect for a picnic, party or lunch pack as it holds well and tastes great at room temperature.

5 garlic cloves, peeled and minced
3¼ cups cooked garbanzo beans (1⅔ cups dried)
⅔ cup warm water
6 tablespoons tahini (available at health food stores, Middle Eastern markets and in the ethnic food section of traditional supermarkets)
¼ cup freshly squeezed lemon juice
1 cup cooked, well-drained spinach
1 tablespoon chopped cilantro

1. Combine all ingredients in a food processor and process until blended.

2. Serve at room temperature and refrigerate any extra.

POWERFOOD HIGHLIGHT
Garlic, garbanzo beans, tahini, lemon juice,
spinach, cilantro

Stuffed Mushrooms

Serves 6

*A*s an appetizer or vegetable side dish, these mushrooms are tasty and satisfying and a guaranteed crowd pleaser whenever they are served. They're easy to assemble, and can be made in advance and reheated. Add a tablespoon of sesame seeds or chopped nuts for extra crunch.

1 pound medium white mushrooms
2 tablespoons butter
⅓ cup minced onion (½ medium onion)
¼ cup minced celery (one 6-inch stalk)
1 teaspoon soy sauce
⅛ teaspoon freshly ground black pepper
1 cup white wine

1. Preheat the oven to 350°F.
2. Wipe the mushrooms clean with damp paper towels. Remove the stems and finely chop them. Set the caps aside.
3. In a large skillet, heat the butter. Sauté the chopped mushroom stems, onion, and celery until the onion becomes transparent (about 10 minutes). Stir in the soy sauce and peppers.
4. Heap the vegetable stuffing in the mushroom caps and arrange in a baking dish.
5. Drizzle the wine over the mushrooms and bake 15 to 20 minutes, until the mushrooms are slightly softened.

POWERFOOD HIGHLIGHT
Mushrooms, onions, celery , nuts and seeds (if used)

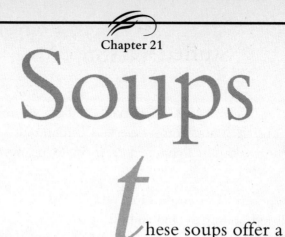

Chapter 21

Soups

*t*hese soups offer a
dazzling rainbow of colors and a potent source of all
nutrients, including phytochemicals. They also present
you with your greatest opportunity for creative
cooking; the variations are limited only by your own
imagination. Enjoy!

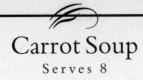

Carrot Soup

Serves 8

*C*arrots and ginger are perfect together and rich in nutrients—especially carotenoids—as well as flavor. Garnish with some chopped green apple for eye-catching appeal.

- 2 tablespoons extra virgin olive oil
- 2 small red onions, peeled and diced
- 1 small leek, green part removed, white part thoroughly cleaned and coarsely chopped
- 2 pounds (approximately 16 medium) carrots, peeled and diced
- 3 tablespoons chopped scallions
- 1 teaspoon minced fresh ginger
- 2½ cups chicken stock or vegetable stock
- ½ cup evaporated skim milk
- Salt and freshly ground black pepper to taste

1. Heat the olive oil in a large saucepan and sauté the onions, leek, carrots, scallion, and ginger over medium heat until tender (about 10 minutes).

2. Add the stock, bring to a boil and simmer for 5 minutes.

3. Remove the soup to a blender and, in batches, purée until smooth.

4. Put the purée back in the saucepan and stir in the skim milk. Reheat but do not boil. Season with salt and pepper to taste.

POWERFOOD HIGHLIGHT
Onions, leek, carrots, scallions, ginger

Kale Soup
Serves 4

*k*ale soup is my favorite fall and winter PowerFood meal-in-a-bowl. Canned beans, drained and rinsed, are a perfectly acceptable time-saving substitute. If some meat would increase your pleasure, add a few slices of low-fat or turkey kielbasa.

¼ cup chick-peas, soaked overnight (½ cup canned)
¼ cup kidney beans, soaked overnight (½ cup canned)
4½ cups chicken stock or vegetable stock
1 cup chopped kale
1 cup diced carrots (about 4 medium carrots)
1 cup julienne strips green cabbage (about ¼ medium cabbage)
1 potato, peeled and diced
1 clove garlic, peeled and minced
2 teaspoons red wine vinegar

1. Rinse the chick-peas and beans and place them in a large saucepan.

2. Cover them with the stock and bring to a boil, uncovered, over high heat. Reduce heat to a simmer. Cook, covered, for 30 minutes.

3. Add the remaining ingredients and cook until the vegetables are tender and the flavors have blended.

POWERFOOD HIGHLIGHT
Chick-peas, kidney beans, kale, carrots, cabbage, garlic

Cream of Mushroom Soup

Serves 8

*f*orget that you ever heard of canned cream of mushroom soup. After you sample this version, convenience won't do. For variety, try your favorite shiitake, oyster, morel, wood ear, or other earthy, flavorful mushroom. A big bowl of this hearty soup, accompanied by salad and a whole grain roll, makes a satisfying lunch or dinner.

2 tablespoons canola oil
2 pounds white mushrooms, sliced
1½ cups diced onions (2 medium onions)
2 potatoes, peeled and cubed
½ cup chopped celery (1 large stalk)
3 cups chicken stock or vegetable stock
¼ cup half-and-half or evaporated skimmed milk
Salt and freshly ground black pepper to taste

1. Heat the canola oil in a large saucepan over medium heat and sauté the mushrooms, onions, potatoes, and celery for 3 or 4 minutes, just until the onions become translucent.

2. Add the stock, bring to a boil, uncovered, and simmer, uncovered, until the vegetables are tender.

3. Transfer the soup to a blender in batches and purée until smooth.

4. Return the soup to the saucepan and whisk in half-and-half or evaporated skimmed milk. Add salt and pepper to taste.

POWERFOOD HIGHLIGHT
Mushrooms, onions, celery

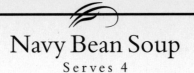

Navy Bean Soup
Serves 4

*n*avy beans are the small, mild, white beans often used in French cooking. In this soup, they are combined with barley and red chard for a complete nutritional PowerFood profile as well as eye appeal. Miso adds a depth of flavor to this recipe.

5 cups vegetable stock
½ cup diced onion
1 (15-ounce) can navy beans, drained and rinsed
1 potato, peeled and diced
2 carrots, thinly sliced
⅔ cup barley
1 cup shredded red chard
2 tablespoons miso
2 tablespoons water

1. Bring ¼ cup of the vegetable stock to a boil in a stockpot. Add the onion and cook for 5 minutes.

2. Add the remaining stock, navy beans, potato, carrots, and barley. Cover and simmer for 30 minutes. (If you are preparing this soup in advance, reheat and continue with Steps 3 to 5).

3. Add the chard, lower the heat, and simmer for a minute or two until the chard wilts. Remove from the heat and set aside.

4. Whisk together the miso and 2 tablespoons of water in a small bowl.

5. Stir into the soup and serve.

POWERFOOD HIGHLIGHT
Onion, navy beans, carrots, barley, red chard, miso

Barbecue Bean Soup

Serves 6

*t*he robust flavor of roasted red peppers makes this soup one of my favorites. It has quite a few ingredients, but the effort is well worth it. The allspice and molasses add sweetness, while the Tabasco gives it just the right barbecue kick. Serve it with Corn Bread (page 317) on a winter day.

1 tablespoon canola oil

1½ cups chopped onions (2 medium onions)

1½ cloves garlic, peeled and coarsely chopped

1 tablespoon chili powder

1 tablespoon cumin

½ teaspoon allspice

⅛ teaspoon ground cloves

2 cups fresh tomatoes, diced, or a 24-ounce can chopped tomatoes, drained

4 cups chicken stock or vegetable stock

2 cups cooked pinto beans (see Note)

1 cup roasted, peeled, chopped red peppers (see Roasted Peppers, page 206, for how to roast and peel peppers)

⅛ cup molasses

2 teaspoons Tabasco

2 teaspoons red wine vinegar

Salt and freshly ground black pepper to taste

1. Heat the oil in a soup pot and cook the onions and garlic over medium heat until the onion is soft and translucent.

2. Stir in the chili powder, cumin, allspice, and cloves, lower the heat, and continue cooking for 2 minutes.

3. Add the tomatoes, chicken stock, pinto beans, red peppers, molasses, and Tabasco and simmer for 2 hours.

4. Just before serving, stir in the vinegar and salt and pepper to taste.

Note: If using fresh beans, they must be soaked overnight

POWERFOOD HIGHLIGHT
Onions, garlic, chili powder, cumin, allspice, cloves, tomatoes, pinto beans, red peppers, molasses, Tabasco

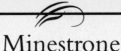

Minestrone
Serves 8

*M*inestrone is the "everything but the kitchen sink" of soups. A little of this and a little of that add up to a quick and easy Italian classic. Once you have tried this recipe, get creative and make your own variations with whatever ingredients you have on hand. A sprinkling of freshly grated Parmesan cheese is a wonderful finishing touch.

1 tablespoon extra virgin olive oil
2 teaspoons minced garlic (4 medium cloves)
1 small onion, diced
2 medium carrots, cut into ½-inch slices
1 medium stalk celery, diced
¼ teaspoon finely chopped fresh thyme
½ teaspoon finely chopped parsley
⅛ teaspoon black pepper
⅛ teaspoon salt
3 cups vegetable stock
½ cup canned, diced tomatoes, drained
½ cup shredded savoy cabbage
3 cups V–8 juice
½ cup cooked red kidney beans
½ cup orzo pasta

1. In a soup pot, heat the oil and sauté the garlic and onion over medium heat until the onion is translucent.

2. Add the carrots, celery, thyme, parsley, black pepper, and salt. Moisten with 3 tablespoons of the stock and cook for 5 minutes.

3. Add the tomatoes, cabbage, V–8 juice, and remaining stock and bring to a boil. Lower the heat, stir in beans and orzo, and simmer, covered, for 20 to 30 minutes.

POWERFOOD HIGHLIGHT:
Garlic, onion, carrots, celery, thyme, parsley, tomatoes, cabbage, V–8 juice, kidney beans

Borscht
Serves 6

*t*his classic Russian soup has such
a rich flavor you won't miss the sour cream borscht typically
contains. It can be served hot or cold with a swirl of plain yogurt
to create a vibrant and tasty combination.

3 medium carrots, chopped
1½ medium onions, diced
4 medium beets, boiled, peeled and chopped
3 cups chicken stock or vegetable stock
1 tablespoon vinegar
6 teaspoons plain nonfat yogurt
Salt and freshly ground black pepper to taste.

1. Place the carrots, onions, and beets in a stockpot. Cover
the vegetables with the stock and simmer over medium heat for
30 minutes.

2. Add the vinegar and stir.

3. Remove the soup from the stockpot and purée it in a blender
in small batches until smooth. Season with salt and pepper.

4. Ladle the soup into bowls and garnish each serving with a
teaspoon of yogurt.

POWERFOOD HIGHLIGHT:
Carrots, onions, beets

Cinnamon Pumpkin Bisque
Serves 6

*t*his slightly sweet soup makes a grand opening to a holiday meal. Experiment with different flavors by substituting other firm-fleshed vegetables like sweet potatoes, buttercup, butternut, acorn, or Hubbard squash.

1 medium onion, diced small
1 tablespoon canola oil
1 clove garlic, peeled and chopped
2 teaspoons ground cinnamon, plus a sprinkling for garnish
2 tablespoons whole wheat flour
5 cups vegetable stock
4 cups cooked pumpkin (canned or fresh)
½ cup soy milk
Salt and freshly ground black pepper to taste.

1. In a large pot, sauté the onion in oil over medium heat until softened. Add the garlic and sauté 2 more minutes. Add cinnamon and flour. Stir until well blended.

2. Slowly pour the stock over the mixture, stirring to combine smoothly. Add the pumpkin and bring to a boil. Lower the heat and simmer, covered, for 20 to 30 minutes.

3. Place in a blender in batches and purée until smooth.

4. Return the soup to the pot and stir in the soy milk. Reheat but do not boil. Season to taste with salt and pepper.

5. Serve sprinkled with additional ground cinnamon.

POWERFOOD HIGHLIGHT
Onion, garlic, cinnamon, whole wheat flour,
pumpkin, soy milk

Cold Blueberry Soup

Serves 8

*C*ool off a hot summer night with this refreshing soup which can serve as the opening act or the grand finale. It's simple to make and festive topped with toasted almonds.

6 cups fresh or frozen blueberries
1 cup pineapple juice
1 teaspoon freshly squeezed lime juice
2 tablespoons sugar
⅛ teaspoon cinnamon
8 teaspoons low-fat plain or lemon yogurt
4 teaspoons slivered almonds

1. Place the blueberries, pineapple juice, lime juice, sugar, and cinnamon in a blender and purée until the consistency is smooth.

2. Serve in soup bowls and garnish each serving with the yogurt and almonds.

POWERFOOD HIGHLIGHT
Blueberries, pineapple juice, lime juice, cinnamon, almonds

Cold Pineapple and Mint Soup

Serves 4

*t*his refreshing and unusual summer fruit soup can start or end your meal. Make sure that your pineapple is ripe and sweet to contrast with the zip and bite of the dry mustard.

1 medium pineapple
2 cups plain nonfat yogurt
½ teaspoon dry mustard
¼ cup fresh chopped mint, plus 4 sprigs for garnish

1. Peel and core the pineapple. Chop the flesh into small dice and set 1 cup of it aside.

2. Combine the remaining pineapple, yogurt, mustard, and chopped mint in a blender and purée until smooth.

3. Serve in bowls garnished with reserved diced pineapple and mint sprigs.

POWERFOOD HIGHLIGHT
Pineapple, mustard, mint

Chapter 22

Salads

*Y*ou won't find iceberg lettuce and Russian dressing here. But you will find some unusual combinations: Sea vegetables, warm salads, whole meals, side salads. The classics are here—four-bean salad and fresh tomatoes with mozzarella—but so are the unexpected. Here's a way to try whole grains in salads, combinations of fruits and vegetables that double the PowerFood punch in a single dish, and alliances of ingredients that are as tasty as they are healthful.

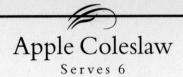

Apple Coleslaw
Serves 6

*t*his tangy coleslaw is quick to prepare, and its beautiful colors and chunky texture make it unique. Serve it with whole grains like Walnut Bulgur (page 272) or Lentil and Brown Rice Casserole (page 278). On its own it makes a great sandwich filling.

1½ cups shredded red cabbage
1½ cups shredded carrots (5 medium carrots)
1 medium onion, thinly sliced
1½ cups diced red apples, skin on (3 apples)
2 teaspoons red wine vinegar
2 teaspoons canola oil
1 tablespoon sugar
1 teaspoon caraway seeds

1. Combine cabbage, carrots, onion, and apples in a large mixing bowl.
2. In a separate bowl, whisk together the vinegar, oil, and sugar.
3. Pour the dressing over the cabbage mixture and sprinkle with caraway seeds. Toss to mix well.
4: Refrigerate 2 to 3 hours before serving.

POWERFOOD HIGHLIGHT
Red cabbage, carrots, onion, apples, caraway seeds

Citrus Asparagus Salad
Serves 4

a trio of citrus tastes heightens and brightens the natural sweet softness of steamed asparagus. This unusual blend of fruits and vegetables combines in minutes. It stands alone as a salad and also lends itself to combining with any variety of grains.

Juice of 1 lemon
Juice of 1 lime
2 tablespoons extra virgin olive oil
1 tablespoon chopped chives
2 tablespoons chopped fresh parsley
2 cups baby greens (mesclun mixture if available)
2 pounds asparagus, cut into 2- to 3-inch pieces and
    steamed until tender
1 grapefruit, peeled and sectioned

1. In a small mixing bowl, combine the lemon and lime juices and grapefruit sections. Add the olive oil, chives, and parsley and mix well.

2. On a serving plate, make a bed of the baby greens and top with the cooked asparagus.

3. Add the grapefruit sections and drizzle on the olive oil-citrus dressing.

POWERFOOD HIGHLIGHT
Lemon juice, lime juice, chives, parsley, greens,
asparagus, grapefruit

Arugula, Radicchio, and Endive Salad

Serves 4

*t*his tangy red, white, and green salad dotted with the orange shreds of carrot can be served at a dinner party or as a surprise change of pace for the everyday family meal.

3 small bunches of arugula, leaves torn into bite-size pieces

1 medium head of radicchio, leaves torn into bite-size pieces

4 heads of Belgian endive, cut crosswise into bite-size pieces

1 carrot, shredded

1 medium tomato, diced

¼ cup extra virgin olive oil

2 tablespoons freshly squeezed lemon juice

1 tablespoon minced fresh chives

Salt and freshly ground black pepper to taste

Tomato wedges (optional)

1. In a large bowl, toss together the arugula, radicchio, Belgian endive, carrot, and tomato.

2. Drizzle the salad with olive oil and lemon juice. Add chives and salt and pepper to taste. Toss well.

3. Serve with tomato wedges and extra lemon if desired.

POWERFOOD HIGHLIGHT

Arugula, radicchio, Belgian endive, carrot, tomato, lemon juice, chives

Arugula and Radicchio Salad
with Sherry Vinaigrette
Serves 4

*t*he mellow sherry vinaigrette softens the bite of arugula and radicchio and makes this a delightful departure from the typical garden salad. Try other vinegars to add a different twist of flavor (for example, raspberry, balsamic, mint, or others of your choice.)

> 2 small bunches of arugula, leaves torn into
>   bite-size pieces
> 1 medium head of radicchio, leaves torn into
>   bite-size pieces
> 1 scallion, diced
> 4 teaspoons red wine vinegar
> 2 teaspoons dry sherry
> 2 tablespoons extra virgin olive oil
> Freshly ground black pepper to taste

1. Place the greens in a salad bowl with the scallion and mix well.

2. In a separate bowl whisk together the vinegar, sherry, and oil. Add to the greens and toss.

3. Add pepper to taste.

POWERFOOD HIGHLIGHT
Arugula, radicchio, scallion

Caesar Salad

Serves 8

*t*his no-egg, low-fat salad is a safe and delicious alternative to the classic Caesar. If topped with grilled chicken strips it becomes a meal in itself.

Dressing
1 cup nonfat cottage cheese
¼ cup buttermilk
1 tablespoon red wine vinegar
3 garlic cloves, peeled and minced
3 small anchovy fillets
¼ cup grated Parmesan cheese
¼ teaspoon freshly ground black pepper
2 tablespoons Dijon mustard
1 teaspoon freshly squeezed lemon juice

2 heads of romaine lettuce, torn into bite-size pieces
2 tablespoons grated Parmesan cheese
Freshly ground black pepper to taste

1. To make the dressing, combine all ingredients in a blender and blend until smooth.

2. To make the salad, combine lettuce, Parmesan, and pepper in a large mixing bowl. Add the dressing and toss well to coat thoroughly.

POWERFOOD HIGHLIGHT
Romaine, garlic, mustard, lemon juice

Napa Cabbage and Mushroom Salad
Serves 6

*t*he feathery napa cabbage and denser red cabbage balance each other nicely. Add the mushrooms and cheese and you have the perfect salad for a luncheon entrée, especially suited for a picnic or a cookout. This recipe also makes a great filling for a toasted sesame bun.

½ head of napa cabbage
½ head of red cabbage
½ pound mushrooms, cleaned and sliced
¼ pound low-fat Swiss cheese
1 tablespoon freshly squeezed lemon juice
1 teaspoon coarse mustard
3 tablespoons extra virgin olive oil
Salt and freshly ground black pepper to taste

1. Cut the cabbages into thin shreds and mix with the mushrooms.

2. Cut the Swiss cheese into thin strips and add to the cabbage and mushroom mixture. Toss well.

3. In a separate bowl, combine the lemon juice, mustard, olive oil, and salt and pepper to taste.

4. Pour the dressing over the salad and toss. Serve.

POWERFOOD HIGHLIGHT
Napa cabbage, red cabbage, mushrooms,
lemon juice, mustard

Cucumber Salad
Serves 6

*C*ucumbers are always refreshing, especially on hot summer days. The coolness of this salad complements curries and other spicy dishes. I love it as a topping for baked potatoes, too.

4 cucumbers, peeled and sliced into ¼-inch rounds
⅓ cup nonfat sour cream or yogurt
1 teaspoon paprika
1 tablespoon freshly squeezed lemon juice
2 tablespoons chopped fresh dill
Salt and freshly ground black pepper to taste

1. Place the cucumber slices in a large sieve and let stand 30 minutes—they will release some of their juices.

2. Pat the cucumber rounds dry with paper towels and place in a salad bowl.

3. In a separate bowl combine the sour cream or yogurt, paprika, lemon juice, dill, and salt and pepper to taste.

4. Gently toss the dressing with the cucumbers; let stand 1 hour and then serve.

POWERFOOD HIGHLIGHT
Cucumbers, paprika, lemon juice, dill

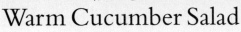

Warm Cucumber Salad
Serves 8

*t*his salad with a sweet and sour dressing is a taste delight, with the added benefit of being heart-healthy and quick to prepare. It's a little more unusual when served warm, and can then double as a vegetable side dish.

6 cucumbers, peeled, cut in half lengthwise, seeded, and sliced

2 onions, thinly sliced

1 clove garlic, peeled and minced

2 tablespoons chopped parsley

½ teaspoon salt

½ teaspoon pepper

½ cup cider vinegar

⅓ cup sugar

¼ cup extra virgin olive oil

1 teaspoon Worcestershire sauce

Mix all the ingredients together in a bowl and toss gently. Warm the salad briefly in a sauté pan and serve. This salad is also tasty served at room temperature.

POWERFOOD HIGHLIGHT
Cucumbers, onions, garlic, parsley

Fennel and Cauliflower Salad

Serves 6

*t*he sweet, aromatic, aniselike flavor of fennel perfectly balances the milder but distinctive taste of cauliflower. This is a great winter salad when lettuce is scarce and variety is lacking. The fennel bulbs (not used in this recipe) are oh so good either braised whole or sliced and added to soups and stews.

1 large head of cauliflower
1 pound fennel stalks, coarsely chopped
⅓ cup extra virgin olive oil
2 tablespoons balsamic vinegar
Salt and freshly ground black pepper to taste

1. Break the cauliflower into florets and steam it until just tender. Cool it in ice immediately after cooking.
2. Put the florets in a salad bowl and add the chopped fennel.
3. In a small bowl, mix together the olive oil and balsamic vinegar. Add salt and pepper to taste.
4. Pour the dressing over the cauliflower and fennel, toss, and serve.

POWERFOOD HIGHLIGHT
Cauliflower, fennel

Fresh Tomatoes with Mozzarella

Serves 4

Summertime, when vine-ripened tomatoes bursting with flavor are available, is the absolute best time to serve this salad. Hothouse tomatoes out of season do not pass muster. I love this salad as a first course or as part of a buffet or picnic.

4 large ripe tomatoes, quartered
¼ pound part-skim mozzarella cheese, cut into small cubes
10 fresh basil leaves, chopped
Salt and freshly ground black pepper to taste
1 teaspoon minced garlic
¼ cup extra virgin olive oil

1. Place the tomatoes, cheese, and basil in a salad bowl and toss gently.
2. Season with salt, pepper, and garlic.
3. Drizzle olive oil over the mixture and let it stand for 1 hour.
4. Serve at room temperature.

POWERFOOD HIGHLIGHT
Tomatoes, basil, garlic

Mango and Watercress Salad with Marinated Chicken

Serves 4

a delightful combination that creates an unusual and satisfying salad entrée.

Marinade
1 tablespoon extra virgin olive oil
2 scallions, chopped
1 clove garlic, peeled and chopped
2 teaspoons chopped fresh parsley
2 (4-ounce) skinless, boneless chicken breasts

Dressing
3 tablespoons extra virgin olive oil
1 shallot, minced
1 tablespoon balsamic vinegar
2 teaspoons finely chopped fresh thyme

½ head of romaine lettuce, shredded
1 head of radicchio, shredded
1 bunch watercress
1 large mango, peeled, pitted, and diced

1. Combine the marinade ingredients in a large shallow bowl. Marinate the chicken at room temperature for 15 to 45 minutes.

2. Whisk together the dressing ingredients in a small mixing bowl.

3. Preheat the broiler to 500°F. Broil the chicken breasts for 10 to 15 minutes, until done, turning once. Let cool slightly.

4. Toss the romaine, radicchio, watercress, and mango in a large bowl. Mix with some of the dressing to coat the greens.

5. Divide the greens and mango salad among 4 bowls. Top each serving with ½ chicken breast and drizzle with remaining dressing.

POWERFOOD HIGHLIGHT
Scallions, garlic, parsley, shallot, thyme, romaine, radicchio, watercress, mango

Fruited Couscous Salad

Serves 8

*t*he exotic tropical fruits called for
in this recipe are now widely available. This salad is so versatile
that you can serve it as a breakfast cereal or as a dinner party dessert
dressed up with a dollop of crème fraîche, or as a side salad
to accompany a fish or chicken entrée. For variety, substitute other
fruits of your choice. Note that this must be made a day ahead.

½ papaya, seeded and diced
½ mango, seeded and diced
4 orange segments, diced
1 kiwi, skinned and diced
1 peach, pitted, skinned, and diced
8 strawberries, diced
¼ cup honey
2 cups cooked couscous (whole wheat couscous if available)
½ cup apple juice
2 tablespoons minced fresh mint

1. Combine all the diced fruits and the honey in a nonreactive
bowl. Add the couscous and mix well.

2. Cover the bowl and let the mixture chill in the refrigerator
overnight.

3. The next day, mix in the apple juice and mint.

4. Serve chilled or at room temperature.

POWERFOOD HIGHLIGHT:
*Papaya, mango, orange, kiwi, peach, strawberries,
couscous, apple juice*

Lemon-zested Couscous
Dinner Salad
Serves 8

*t*his salad's claim to fame is that it serves as a complete vegetarian main dish, especially on hot summer days, and is the only accompaniment you need with a chicken, fish, or lamb entrée. Season your meat with lemon zest, fresh rosemary, and garlic if you like, and grill.

1 tablespoon extra virgin olive oil
4 cups shredded vegetables (carrots, cabbage, beets, zucchini, summer squash, or others of choice)
Grated zest of 2 lemons
1 tablespoon freshly squeezed lemon juice
1½ tablespoons chopped fresh parsley
½ teaspoon chopped fresh rosemary
1 cup cooked couscous (whole wheat couscous if available)

1. Put the oil in a nonstick skillet and place over medium heat.

2. Add all the vegetables (see Note) and cook, uncovered, until tender. Transfer the vegetables to a mixing bowl.

3. Dress the vegetables with the lemon zest, lemon juice, parsley and rosemary. Set aside and let cool.

4. Combine the couscous with the cooked, dressed vegetables, mix gently, and serve at room temperature.

Note: If using beets, turnips, or rutabagas, you need to parboil them before sautéing.

POWERFOOD HIGHLIGHT
Shredded vegetables, lemon zest, lemon juice, parsley, rosemary, couscous

Buckwheat Salad

Serves 8

*b*uckwheat is a tasty grain that makes a hearty salad for any occasion. I especially love it served warm. The addition of chick-peas or other favorite beans make it substantial enough to merit a starring role as a vegetarian main course.

> 4 cups vegetable stock
> 2 cups buckwheat groats (kasha)
> 1 cup chopped cucumber, skin on (1 medium cucumber)
> 1 cup minced fresh parsley
> 2 tablespoons red wine vinegar
> ⅓ cup extra virgin olive oil

1. Place the stock in a large saucepan and bring to a boil. Add the buckwheat and cook, covered, over medium heat until tender and all liquid is absorbed, approximately 10 minutes.

2. Set it aside to cool.

3. Combine the cucumber, cooled buckwheat, and parsley in a nonreactive bowl and toss well.

4. Whisk the olive oil and vinegar together. Drizzle over the salad and toss gently to coat. Let stand for 1 hour before serving.

POWERFOOD HIGHLIGHT
Buckwheat, cucumber, parsley

Brown Rice Salad
Serves 8

*S*erve this unusual grain and vegetable salad on a bed of greens and garnish with sesame seeds and sprigs of watercress. It is easy to prepare and can be made up to two or three days ahead of time. If you make it in advance, keep it refrigerated until needed, but leave enough time for the salad to reach room temperature to bring out the flavor.

2 cups long-grain brown rice
4 cups vegetable stock
¼ teaspoon sea salt
1 cup finely diced carrots, (3 medium carrots)
1 cup finely diced celery (½ stalk)
2 tablespoons brown rice miso

1. Place all the ingredients in a large saucepan and bring to a boil. Cook, covered, over low heat for 45 minutes.

2. Remove the rice mixture and pack in a mold sprayed with nonstick vegetable spray.

3. Chill for at least 2 hours.

4. Unmold and serve at room temperature.

POWERFOOD HIGHLIGHT
Brown rice, carrots, celery, miso

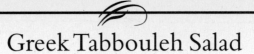

Greek Tabbouleh Salad
Serves 6

*t*his quick and easy Mediterra-
nean cracked wheat salad is a whole grain side dish that also makes
a wonderful pita pocket sandwich filling. My favorite sandwich
is a pita pocket spread with a few spoons of Spinach Hummus
(page 207) and filled with this tabbouleh salad.

3 cups bulgur (cracked wheat)
3 scallions, chopped
2 large tomatoes, diced
1 bunch parsley, chopped fine
2 tablespoons finely chopped mint
¼ cup extra virgin olive oil
½ cup freshly squeezed lemon juice
Pinch salt

1. Combine the bulgur and 6 cups water in a large saucepan.
Bring to a boil, reduce heat, and cook, covered, for 10 to 15 minutes.
Drain, place in a bowl, and let bulgur cool.

2. Add all the remaining ingredients and mix well.

3. Serve at room temperature. This salad looks especially attractive placed on a leaf of red-edged lettuce.

POWERFOOD HIGHLIGHT
Bulgur, scallions, tomatoes, parsley, mint, lemon juice

Hijiki Tossed Salad

Serves 6

*I*f you want to reap the health benefits of sea vegetables, dare to try this rather typical garden salad with the added touch of the sea. Hijiki is one of the stronger flavored sea vegetables. A mere one-quarter cup adds a tremendous amount of flavor. It is available dried in Asian markets or health food stores. The different textures and colors and variety of flavors will delight all your senses.

¼ cup dried hijiki
½ head of Bibb lettuce, chopped
½ head of romaine lettuce, chopped
1 medium cucumber, peeled and thinly sliced
½ cup alfalfa sprouts
2 or 3 radishes, sliced
1 small onion, sliced
2 tomatoes, cut into quarters

1. Soak hijiki in water for 4 to 5 minutes and set aside.

2. Toss all the greens and other vegetables in a large salad bowl and add the hijiki. Mix well.

3. Serve with Miso Vinaigrette (page 300) or other dressing of your choice.

POWERFOOD HIGHLIGHT
Hijiki, Bibb, romaine, cucumber, alfalfa sprouts, radishes, onion, tomatoes

Udon and Vegetable Salad

Serves 8

*P*erk up your taste buds and your pasta with the combination of sesame, scallion, tamari, and red pepper flakes. The Asian theme of the sauce works best with udon, but fresh linguine is a good second choice.

2 packages udon noodles
3 medium carrots, shredded
4 scallions, chopped
1 red pepper, cut into strips
¼ cup sesame oil
¼ cup tamari
⅛ teaspoon red pepper flakes

1. Cook the noodles according to the manufacturer's instructions. Drain, rinse, and refrigerate until chilled.
2. In a large bowl, combine all the remaining ingredients.
3. Add the noodles and toss, mixing well. Serve chilled.

POWERFOOD HIGHLIGHT
Udon noodles, carrots, scallions, red pepper

Four-Bean Salad
Serves 8

*t*his traditional four-bean salad is dressed up with black beans and red peppers.. If you're using canned beans, rinse them and drain.

2 medium-size sweet red peppers
¼ pound fresh green beans, trimmed and snapped in two
1 small onion, thinly sliced
1 cup cooked and drained navy beans
1 cup cooked and drained black beans
1 cup cooked and drained kidney beans
¼ cup extra virgin olive oil
¼ cup freshly squeezed lemon juice
1 teaspoon sugar
2 tablespoons minced fresh parsley
Salt and freshly ground black pepper to taste

1. Preheat the broiler to 500°F.
2. Place the red peppers on the broiler pan and broil them, turning three times, until they are charred on all sides. Remove them to a bowl and cover with plastic wrap. Leave for 10 minutes (this will make the peppers easy to peel).
3. Peel and core the peppers over a small bowl to catch and reserve the juice. Discard the seeds and then slice lengthwise into strips.
4. In a small pan, steam the green beans until they are crisp-tender. Rinse and refresh the beans under cold water.
5. In a large, nonreactive bowl, combine the onion, navy beans, black beans, and kidney beans. Add the red peppers, their reserved juice, and the green beans. Toss gently with olive oil and lemon juice.
6. Sprinkle with the sugar, parsley, salt, and black pepper. Stir until mixed well.
7. Cover and chill for at least 2 hours before serving.

POWERFOOD HIGHLIGHT
Red peppers, green beans, onion, navy beans, black beans, kidney beans, lemon juice, parsley

PowerFoods

Chapter 23

Vegetable Side Dishes

*t*his chapter on vegeta-
bles exemplifies the PowerFoods program. Eating

vegetables is the prerequisite for good health,

and particularly for maintaining a healthy weight.

For those who think they don't like vegetables—

who still confuse them with the overcooked lumps

they had to eat in childhood before they were allowed

dessert—these recipes should be a revelation. For

those who already love vegetables, these "side" dishes

can be main dishes for any meal, anytime. Two

or three of these together pack all the nutrient and

phytochemical power that food has to offer, and they

should satisfy every appetite and every taste.

Beets with Tarragon

Serves 6

*R*uby red beets sprinkled with snippets of tarragon make a marvelous marriage of taste and eye appeal. The optional flavor-intensifying step (see Note) is worth the extra minute or two. For a different appearance, but just as attractive, the beets can be sliced instead of cubed.

12 small beets
1 tablespoon sugar
1 tablespoon snipped fresh tarragon
Salt and freshly ground black pepper to taste
2 tablespoons butter or 2 tablespoons tarragon
    vinegar (optional)

1. Boil the beets in lightly salted water until they are tender, about 45 minutes.

2. Peel the beets and cut them into cubes.

3. In a small bowl, mix together the sugar, tarragon, salt, and pepper. Toss with the beets.

4. Serve warm or chilled.

Note: To intensify the flavor, sauté the cubed seasoned beets in either butter or tarragon vinegar.

POWERFOOD HIGHLIGHT
Beets, tarragon

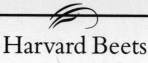

Harvard Beets
Serves 6

*t*hese sweet and sour beets with the clinging sauce deliver a mouthful of flavor with every bite. The recipe is a classic.

6 medium beets
¼ cup cider vinegar
¼ cup brown sugar
2 teaspoons cornstarch
¼ teaspoon ground cloves
1 cup sliced onions

1. Boil the beets in lightly salted water until tender. Drain the beets and reserve their cooking water. Peel and cube or slice the beets.

2. Combine the beet water and additional water if necessary to make 1 cup. Add vinegar, brown sugar, cornstarch, cloves, and onions.

3. Bring the mixture to a boil, stirring constantly until juice thickens into a light syrup.

4. Remove the sauce from the heat and drizzle it over the beets, coating them with the sauce; add more sauce if necessary.

5. Serve hot or at room temperature.

POWERFOOD HIIGHLIGHT
Beets, cloves, onions

Sweet and Spiced Baby Carrots

S e r v e s 6

*b*aby carrots glazed with spices that enhance their inner sweetness are truly a taste treat. This is a classic side dish, but also makes a wonderful hors d'oeuvre, appetizer, or even a between-meal snack. It's tastier and lots healthier than candy.

2 pounds whole baby carrots, scrubbed and peeled
2 tablespoons unsalted butter
3 tablespoons dark brown sugar
½ teaspoon ground ginger
½ teaspoon cinnamon
½ teaspoon allspice

1. Steam the carrots until tender in a large saucepan so that they are not crowded, about 10 to 12 minutes. Remove them from the heat and set aside.

2. In a large saucepan, melt the butter. Add the brown sugar and seasonings.

3. Toss the carrots with the butter, sugar, and seasoning mixture.

4. Cook 3 to 5 minutes over medium heat, stirring gently, until the carrots have caramelized.

5. Remove from the heat immediately and serve.

POWERFOOD HIGHLIGHT
Carrots, ginger, cinnamon, allspice

Summer Squash Stir-Fry
with Tomatoes
Serves 4

*S*ummer squash can be yellow or green, and they are always best when plucked fresh from your garden or the local farm stand. This recipe is a wonderful side dish and it also fits into the category of "toppers." Adorn your pasta, potatoes, whole grain toasted garlic bread, or even a fish fillet with this juicy, flavorful blend. If a sprinkle of Parmesan appeals to you, go for it.

1 tablespoon canola oil
1 cup diced ripe tomatoes
3 cups 1-inch cubes mixed summer squash
1 garlic clove, peeled and minced
¼ cup soy sauce or tamari

1. Heat the oil in a medium-size skillet. Add the vegetables and sauté until tender.

2. Add the garlic and soy sauce, and stir to coat the vegetables well. Continue to cook 5 more minutes.

POWERFOOD HIGHLIGHT
Tomatoes, summer squash, garlic

Pattypan Squash Creole

Serves 8

*b*aby pattypans are the tenderest and best squash for this recipe. It is remarkably attractive to present the whole squash with the colorful red, green, and black-flecked vegetable medley. The combination of herbs and Cajun seasoning will spice up any meal.

4 pounds mixed baby pattypan squash
¼ cup extra virgin olive oil
1 medium onion, sliced
2 garlic cloves, peeled and minced
½ cup pitted kalamata olives
1 green pepper, seeded and diced
4 fresh tomatoes, quartered and seeded
1 tablespoon chopped fresh basil
1 tablespoon chopped fresh oregano
1 teaspoon Cajun seasoning spice
Salt and freshly ground black pepper to taste

1. Preheat the oven to 350°F.

2. Place the squash in a large casserole dish. Pour olive oil over it and toss to coat.

3. Toss the squash together with all remaining ingredients, cover, and bake for 45 to 60 minutes or until tender.

4. If desired, uncover and continue to cook for 10 to 15 minutes to reduce the amount of liquid in the casserole.

POWERFOOD HIGHLIGHT
Pattypan squash, onion, garlic, olives, green pepper, tomatoes, basil, oregano

Spaghetti Squash with Pine Nuts
Serves 4 to 6

Spaghetti squash is fun to prepare and even more fun to eat. It's a vegetable version of pasta, this one with pesto. The flavor of basil and texture of toasted pine nuts are the perfect partners for this mild-mannered squash.

¼ cup pine nuts, toasted
2 medium spaghetti squash
2 tablespoons butter
½ cup chopped fresh basil
1 teaspoon salt
1 teaspoon freshly ground black pepper

1. Preheat the oven to 375°F.
2. Spread the pine nuts on a baking sheet and toast them until lightly browned, watching carefully to be sure they do not burn. Remove them from the oven and set aside to cool.
3. Liberally prick the spaghetti squash with a fork to prevent them from bursting when baking. Place them on a baking sheet and bake 45 minutes to 1 hour. Remove from the oven and set aside to cool.
4. Cut the squash in half lengthwise, scoop out the seeds, and discard.
5. With a fork, comb all the strands of flesh from each half section and discard shells.
6. In a large skillet, melt the butter over low heat, add the squash strands, and toss while reheating. Stir in the pine nuts, basil, salt, and pepper.
6. Serve hot.

POWERFOOD HIGHLIGHT
Pine nuts, squash, basil

Citrus Butternut Squash

Serves 8

*t*angy orange and pineapple, zippy ginger, and sweet butternut squash come alive with the crunch of pistachio. Spruce up holiday time or anytime with this daring departure from the more traditional baked squash.

- 2 large butternut squash, peeled, seeded, and diced
- 3 tablespoons molasses
- 2 tablespoons brown sugar
- ½ teaspoon salt
- ⅛ teaspoon freshly grated ginger
- ¼ cup canned crushed pineapple
- ¼ cup roughly chopped pistachio nuts
- 1 cup orange juice, more or less, depending on consistency desired

1. Place the squash in a saucepan and add water to cover halfway.
2. Cook the squash over medium heat until soft. Drain the water and then mash the squash pieces with a fork.
3. Stir in the molasses, brown sugar, salt, ginger, crushed pineapple, and nuts.
4. Gradually add orange juice and stir until the desired consistency is reached.

POWERFOOD HIGHLIGHT
Butternut squash, ginger, pineapple, pistachio nuts, orange juice

Maple-baked Winter Squash

Serves 8

*M*aple syrup adds a sweet touch and delicate glaze to this hearty squash. Apple cider adds a unique flavor and additional moisture if it is used instead of butter.

    4 acorn squash
    2 tablespoons butter or 2 tablespoons apple cider
    1 cup pure maple syrup
    1 teaspoon ground cinnamon

1. Preheat the oven to 375°F.

2. Wash and cut each acorn squash into 4 wedges. Remove the seeds and place the squash in a large baking dish.

3. In a saucepan, melt the butter (or heat the apple cider) and add the maple syrup, stirring over low heat until the ingredients are combined.

4. Pour the syrup over the squash and then sprinkle with cinnamon.

5. Bake 45 to 60 minutes, basting the squash with the syrup from the bottom of the baking dish every 15 to 20 minutes, until the squash is tender.

POWERFOOD HIGHLIGHT
Acorn squash, apple cider, cinnamon

Honeyed Sweet Potatoes

Serves 6

*t*hese sweet potatoes satisfy like candy. They are a delicious, nutritious treat that's a cinch to make. I recommend them for holidays, family meals, and special snacks.

6 medium sweet potatoes, peeled
½ cup honey
1–2 teapoons freshly ground cinnamon

1. Cook the sweet potatoes in boiling salted water until they are barely tender. Drain and let them cool.

2. Preheat the oven to 350°F.

3. Cut the potatoes crosswise into ¼-inch slices. Place the sliced potatoes in a casserole sprayed with nonstick vegetable spray. Drizzle with honey, sprinkle with cinnamon, and bake for 35 minutes, basting the sweet potatoes until they are nicely glazed.

POWERFOOD HIGHLIGHT
Sweet potatoes, cinnamon

Sweet-and-Sour Red Cabbage
Serves 8

*t*his is my all-time favorite cabbage recipe. It is easy to prepare after you get past shredding the cabbage. The unique flavor of juniper berries is a delightful addition, but if they're not on hand, don't worry. (The caraway seeds, however, are indispensable.) This recipe freezes well and I always have it on hand for a quick company dish. My friends share my enthusiasm.

2 tablespoons canola oil
1 medium onion, coarsely chopped
¼ cup brown sugar
1 teaspoon salt
½ teaspoon black pepper
1 teaspoon allspice
¼ teaspoon cloves
1 apple, peeled, cored, and cubed
1 to 2 pounds red cabbage, finely shredded
½ cup red wine vinegar
½ cup juniper berries
1 tablespoon caraway seeds

1. Heat the oil in a large skillet over medium heat. Add the onion and sauté until golden brown, about 5 minutes.

2. Add the sugar, seasonings, apple, and shredded cabbage, stirring to combine well. Add ¼ cup boiling water, cover, and simmer for 1 hour, adding more water if necessary to keep moistened.

3. Add the vinegar, juniper berries, and caraway seeds. Simmer for another 10 to 15 minutes. Serve hot.

POWERFOOD HIGHLIGHT
Onion, allspice, cloves, apple, red cabbage, juniper berries, caraway seeds

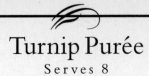

Turnip Purée

Serves 8

*M*ashed turnips crowned with sautéed onions is admittedly an unusual presentation. Its delicious flavor will win you over, and, I hope, will increase your use of this delicious root vegetable. This recipe triggers my imagination, and I have added mashed potato or mashed carrots to the turnip mixture with great success. In addition, you can substitute for the white turnips the stronger-flavored large yellow turnips called rutabagas.

6 medium white turnips, peeled and chopped
Salt and pepper to taste
2 teaspoons unsalted butter
2 medium onions, cut in half crosswise and thinly sliced
2 tablespoons fresh lemon juice
¼ cup chopped fresh parsley
1 teaspoon caraway seeds

1. Place the turnips and a dash of salt in a large pot and cover with water. Bring the water to a boil and cook until the turnips are tender.

2. Melt the butter in a skillet over medium heat and sauté the onions with the lemon juice and chopped parsley for 10 minutes, or until the onions are transparent and soft.

3. Drain and mash the turnips. Stir in the caraway seeds, salt, and pepper and transfer to a serving dish.

4. Pour the onion mixture on top and serve immediately.

POWERFOOD HIGHLIGHT
Turnips, onions, lemon juice, parsley, caraway seeds

Roasted Red Peppers and
Brussels Sprouts

Serves 8

*b*russels sprouts—you either love them or hate them. I love them this way, mingled with roasted red peppers and baked into sweetness. If you're unsure of your position on brussels spouts, I recommend that you give this recipe a try.

2 red peppers, halved and seeded
½ tablespoon extra virgin olive oil
1½ pounds (3 cups) cooked brussels sprouts
1 clove garlic, peeled and minced
Salt and freshly ground black pepper to taste
1 tablespoon minced fresh dill

1. Preheat the oven to 350°F.

2. Place the peppers on a cookie sheet and brush with the oil. Bake for 30 minutes. Remove the peppers from the oven, let cool, and then peel and seed. Cut the peppers into ¼-inch strips.

3. Place the cooked brussels sprouts in a glass or ceramic baking dish. Stir in the pepper strips. Season with garlic, salt, and pepper, tossing to mix well.

4. Bake uncovered for 10 minutes and garnish with fresh dill.

POWERFOOD HIGHLIGHT
Red peppers, brussels sprouts, garlic, dill

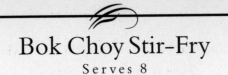

Bok Choy Stir-Fry
Serves 8

*S*weet and pungent from the two varieties of onion, this stir-fry is a fast, delicious way to power up your vegetable intake. Even your kids will love it. For nutritional completeness and to continue the Asian theme, you can add cubed tofu and serve over rice.

- 1 tablespoon sesame oil
- 1 large head of bok choy, cleaned and chopped into 1-inch pieces
- 2 medium red onions, cut into thin strips
- 2 medium yellow onions, cut into thin strips
- 1 small clove garlic, peeled and minced
- 1 tablespoon soy sauce

1. Heat a wok or skillet and swirl in the sesame oil.
2. Add the bok choy, onions, and garlic and stir-fry over high heat 3 to 5 minutes, or until the vegetables are tender.
3. Stir in the soy sauce and serve immediately.

POWERFOOD HIGHLIGHT
Bok choy, onions, garlic

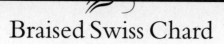

Braised Swiss Chard
Serves 4 to 6

*t*his underappreciated but delicious vegetable is the perfect accompaniment to Barley Risotto (page 275), Brown Rice Pilaf (page 276), Walnut Bulgur (page 272), or other whole-grain casseroles. Swiss chard has become widely available, so look for it in your supermarket and try this recipe for a pleasant taste sensation.

> 3 tablespoons extra virgin olive oil
> 2 garlic cloves, peeled and chopped
> 1 teaspoon dried rosemary
> 2 pounds (approximately 2 bunches) Swiss chard, washed and coarsely chopped
> Salt and freshly ground black pepper to taste
> ¼ cup white wine

1. Heat the olive oil in a large sauté pan over low heat. Sauté the garlic and rosemary for about 2 minutes, just until the garlic begins to release its flavor but before it turns golden.

2. Add the Swiss chard, salt, and pepper. Cover and cook for 15 minutes over low heat.

3. Add the wine and continue to cook over low heat 10 minutes longer. Serve immediately.

POWERFOOD HIGHLIGHT
Swiss chard, garlic, rosemary

Steamed Cauliflower
with Chive Butter
Serves 8

*P*repared this way, cauliflower develops a succulent flavor. A touch of chive adds taste and color. For a special look, steam the cauliflower whole, drizzle with chive butter and serve it surrounded by Sautéed Porcini Mushrooms (page 262).

2 heads of cauliflower
2 tablespoons butter
¼ cup chopped fresh chives
1 teaspoon freshly squeezed lemon juice
Salt and freshly ground black pepper to taste

1. Wash the cauliflower and break it into florets. Steam until tender, approximately 15 minutes.

2. In a small saucepan, melt the butter over low heat and combine with the remaining ingredients.

3. Drizzle the chive butter over the cauliflower florets. Serve warm.

POWERFOOD HIGHLIGHT
Cauliflower, chives, lemon juice

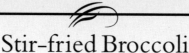

Stir-fried Broccoli

Serves 6

*t*his is only one of many ways to serve broccoli, the workhorse of the cruciferous vegetable group. A stir-fry is always fast, always delicious, and lends itself to endless variations limited only by your imagination. I like to add cubed tofu or chicken strips and serve it with brown rice for a complete meal.

2 heads of fresh broccoli
2 tablespoons dark sesame oil
2 scallions, cut in 1-inch sections (include both white
    and green parts)
1½ teaspoons soy sauce
½ teaspoon sugar
2 tablespoons sesame seeds

1. Wash the broccoli and break it into small florets with some of the stem attached. Peel the larger stems and cut into ½-inch rounds.

2. Heat a wok or skillet over high heat for 30 seconds and swirl in the oil.

3. Briskly stir-fry the broccoli florets, broccoli stems, and scallions for 4 to 5 minutes or until tender. Combine the soy sauce and sugar and add to the broccoli.

4. Cook over medium heat for another 10 minutes, adding a little water if necessary to steam and soften the broccoli.

5. Toss with sesame seeds. Serve immediately.

POWERFOOD HIGHLIGHT
Broccoli, scallions, sesame seeds

Creamy Broccoli Casserole

Serves 4 as an Entrée or 8 as a Side Dish

*A*lthough this recipe is a mix of fresh and processed ingredients (and not as low in fat as I usually recommend), it is so creamy, cheesy, and convenient that I just had to include it. It freezes well and you can defrost it in minutes in a microwave oven and have it ready in a flash. It is a comfort food, loved by kids (and their parents) of all ages.

2 heads fresh broccoli, broken into florets and steamed
1 (8-ounce) can cream of broccoli soup
½ cup bran flakes cereal, crushed
¼ cup grated Romano cheese
Freshly ground black pepper to taste

1. Preheat the oven to 350°F.
2. Place the steamed broccoli florets in a casserole.
3. Pour the cream of broccoli soup over the broccoli. Sprinkle bran flakes and cheese over the mixture. Add pepper to taste.
4. Bake the broccoli for 15 to 20 minutes or until the topping is golden brown.

POWERFOOD HIGHLIGHT
Broccoli, bran flakes

Spinach and Mushroom Stir-Fry

Serves 4

*S*oy and sesame always perk up stir-fried greens. With mushrooms and garlic, this is an ideal vegetable accompaniment to a whole-grain, fish, or chicken entrée.

3 tablespoons dark sesame oil
2 garlic cloves, peeled and minced
2 cups sliced fresh mushrooms
2 pounds fresh spinach, washed, spun dry, and chopped
1 teaspoon sugar
¼ cup soy sauce

1. Place wok over high heat for 30 seconds. Swirl in the oil.

2. Briskly stir-fry the garlic until lightly browned, about 30 seconds. Add the mushrooms and cook for another 10 minutes or until the mushrooms are tender.

3. Add the spinach to the wok and cook another 2 to 3 minutes, until the spinach wilts.

4. Combine sugar and soy sauce and stir into spinach and mushroom mixture. Serve immediately.

POWERFOOD HIGHLIGHT
Garlic, mushrooms, spinach

Sweet–and–Sour Onions

Serves 4

*E*legant small white onions glazed with a tangy caramelized sauce are the perfect accompaniment to a chicken, fish, or whole-grain entrée. Add braised or stir-fried greens for nutritional completeness and eye-appealing color.

2 pounds small white onions
2 tablespoons butter
¼ cup brown sugar
¼ cup red wine vinegar
Salt and pepper to taste

1. In a large saucepan, bring 4 cups of lightly salted water to a boil.

2. Cross-cut the root ends, blanch quickly in boiling water, then peel the onions and boil them until tender, about 15 minutes.

3. Melt the butter in a large skillet over medium heat. Add the whole onions and sauté them for 5 to 10 minutes, turning them frequently, until they begin to brown.

4. Add the brown sugar and stir until it melts, about 1 or 2 minutes.

5. Add the vinegar and salt and pepper. Cook until the sauce thickens and coats the onions.

POWERFOOD HIGHLIGHT
Onions

Burgundy Mushrooms and Onions

Serves 6

*b*urgundy wine and butter create
a deep and very rich taste sensation. The mushrooms and onions
meld into a mouth-watering accompaniment to your occasional
steak or more frequent baked potato. Don't be afraid of the butter:
It works out to 1 teaspoon per serving—about 45 calories and
5 grams of fat.

> 2 tablespoons butter
> 2 pounds sliced fresh mushrooms
> 1 large onion, sliced
> 1 clove garlic, peeled and minced
> ⅛ teaspoon salt
> ⅛ teaspoon freshly ground black pepper
> ¼ cup burgundy wine

1. Melt the butter in a sauté pan and cook the mushrooms
and onion over medium heat until the onion is translucent, about
5 to 7 minutes.

2. Season with garlic, salt, and pepper. Continue to cook over
medium heat for 5 to 10 minutes more, until the mushrooms are
tender and the liquid is absorbed.

3. Stir in the burgundy wine and cook uncovered over medium
heat for 2 or 3 minutes longer.

POWERFOOD HIGHLIGHT
Mushrooms, onion, garlic

Sautéed Porcini Mushrooms

Serves 8

*W*e've all grown up with the basic, white button mushroom. The robust flavor of some of our more exotic mushrooms will, I hope, inspire us to use them more and more. For variety, substitute others, such as portobello, shiitake, cremini, or morels. They are really special and fortunately now widely available.

2 tablespoons extra virgin olive oil
2 garlic cloves, peeled and minced
2 pounds whole porcini mushrooms
¼ cup sherry

1. Preheat the oven to 350°F.
2. Combine the oil, garlic, and mushrooms in a skillet with an ovenproof handle.
3. Sauté uncovered over medium heat for about 5 minutes or until the mushrooms begin to release their juices. Drizzle with sherry.
4. Place the skillet in the oven, cover, and bake for 15 to 20 minutes or until the mushrooms are tender.
5. Serve hot.

POWERFOOD HIGHLIGHT
Garlic, mushrooms

Lentils with Nori

Serves 4 as an Entrée or 8 as a Side Dish

*S*ubstantial lentils mingled with milder seaweed (nori) strips cook into a stewlike consistency. Topped with the crunch of toasted sesame seeds and served over brown rice, this dish fulfills all taste and nutritional requirements. When using it as a main course, top with steamed vegetables of your choice. (Mine for this recipe would be carrots.)

> 2 cups lentils, rinsed and picked over
> 2 sheets nori, soaked until softened and cut into strips
> ½ teaspoon sea salt
> 2 cloves garlic, peeled and minced
> 2 teaspoons miso paste
> 2 tablespoons toasted sesame seeds

1. Combine all ingredients except sesame seeds with 6 cups of water in a saucepan. Cover and cook over low heat for 30 to 45 minutes.
2. Sprinkle with toasted sesame seeds.

POWERFOOD HIGHLIGHT
Lentils, nori, garlic, miso paste, sesame seeds

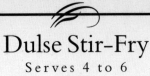

Dulse Stir-Fry

Serves 4 to 6

*f*or those with adventurous palates and time to track down these varied ingredients, this recipe is a real treasure. It is actually a pleasant and easy way to incorporate sea vegetables into your life.

2 tablespoons dark sesame oil
2 ounces dried dulse, soaked until softened, and sliced
3 carrots, peeled and cut into thin 2-inch-long sticks
3 parsnips, peeled and cut into thin sticks
1 medium daikon radish, peeled and cut into thin sticks
½ cup water chestnuts, sliced
1 tablespoon tamari

1. Place a wok over high heat for 30 seconds. Swirl in the sesame oil. Add the dulse and vegetables. Sauté 10 to 12 minutes, stirring constantly to avoid burning. Remove from the wok to a serving bowl.

2. Season with tamari and serve immediately.

POWERFOOD HIGHLIGHT
Dulse, carrots, parsnips, daikon

Marinated Wakame and Zucchini Sticks

Serves 8

*t*his recipe gives basic zucchini an exotic twist. It also makes an interesting sandwich filling or appetizer accompanied by crisp crackers. Pickled ginger is always available in Asian markets but may also be found in your health food store. Ask for it.

4 zucchini, cut in 2-inch matchsticks
2 ounces wakame, soaked until softened
1 tablespoon chopped pickled ginger
1 teaspoon sea salt
1 teaspoon tamari

1. Bring a pot of water to a boil. Add the zucchini sticks and when the water returns to a boil, remove the zucchini. Rinse with cold water and drain.

2. Rinse the wakame after it has been soaked and slice into ½-inch strips.

3. Place all the ingredients in a bowl. Toss them to combine well. Cover and place in the refrigerator overnight.

4. Bring to room temperature before serving.

POWERFOOD HIGHLIGHT
Zucchini, wakame, ginger

Wakame with Parsnips and Carrots

Serves 4

*E*arth and sea are combined in this root vegetable and seaweed recipe. The flavor of each complements the other. Served over brown rice, millet, or quinoa, it is truly a meal in a bowl, and I know several people who have taken to it for breakfast. I love it as a light supper entrée.

  2 ounces dried wakame, soaked until softened, rinsed, and drained
  2 parsnips, peeled and diced
  2 carrots, peeled and diced
  1 tablespoon tamari

1. Place the parsnips, carrots, and wakame in a saucepan.
2. Cover with 2 cups water and bring to a boil. Reduce heat and simmer, partially covered, for 15 to 20 minutes.
3. Drain the water. Place the vegetables in a bowl and toss with tamari.

POWERFOOD HIGHLIGHT
Wakame, parsnips, carrots

Potatoes with Vegetable Salsa
Serves 4

a powerhouse of PowerFoods, this recipe answers the perennial question "What do I put on top of my potato?" This dish works well as an entrée, served with a salad. For a change, serve half of a potato as an appetizer. Substitute a sweet potato for extra nutrition.

4 Idaho or russet baking potatoes
1 tablespoon extra virgin olive oil
½ red pepper, seeded and diced
½ yellow pepper, seeded and diced
½ green pepper, seeded and diced
1 medium red onion, diced
1 clove garlic, peeled and chopped
4 plum tomatoes, diced
1 teaspoon chopped cilantro
1 tablespoon freshly squeezed lime juice
¼ cup Parmesan cheese

1. Preheat the oven to 400°F.
2. Bake the potatoes for 50 to 60 minutes, until soft. (Leave the oven on.) Cut in half.
3. Heat the olive oil in a skillet over medium heat and sauté the peppers, onion, and garlic until softened.
4. Add the plum tomatoes, cilantro, and lime juice to the pepper mixture. Cook until the tomatoes are heated through.
5. Pour the salsa over the potato halves, sprinkle with Parmesan cheese, and return them to the oven until the cheese is lightly browned, about 5 minutes.

POWERFOOD HIGHLIGHT
Red, yellow, green peppers; red onion, garlic, tomatoes, cilantro, lime juice

Southern Succotash

Serves 4

*S*uccotash always includes corn and beans. Okra adds the Southern flair, tomatoes add color and flavor, and it all combines into a mixed vegetable casserole that is perfect for an informal buffet.

3 large tomatoes, peeled, seeded, and chopped
½ pound okra, fresh or frozen
¼ cup coarsely chopped celery
½ pound frozen lima beans
¼ cup vegetable stock
½ pound frozen corn kernels
Salt and freshly ground black pepper to taste

1. In a saucepan, combine the tomatoes, okra, and celery. Simmer, covered, over medium heat for 5 minutes.

2. Add the lima beans and vegetable stock. Simmer for 10 minutes more.

3. Add the corn and simmer 5 more minutes or until all the vegetables are tender and heated through.

4. Season with salt and pepper. Serve hot.

POWERFOOD HIGHLIGHT
Tomatoes, okra, celery, lima beans, corn

Stuffed Tomatoes with Rice and Pecans

Serves 6

*i*n tomato season, this recipe is perfect as a light vegetable entrée for lunch or dinner or as a substantial side dish to complement grilled fish. The chopped pecans are an essential taste and texture component.

6 large tomatoes
1 cup brown rice
½ cup chopped pecans
Salt and pepper to taste
2 cloves garlic, peeled and minced
3 cups chicken stock or vegetable stock
3 tablespoons finely chopped fresh parsley

1. Preheat the oven to 450°F.

2. Cut off the stem ends of the tomatoes; scoop out and discard the seeds and central flesh, forming large cups. Place cups upside down to drain.

3. Rinse the rice. Bring 3 cups of water to a boil in a saucepan. Add the rice and cook uncovered for 15 minutes.

4. Drain the rice in a colander as you would pasta. It should be a little firm. Stir the pecans into the rice.

5. Arrange the tomato cups in a baking dish. Sprinkle with salt and pepper and fill with the rice mixture.

6. Over the rice, sprinkle the chopped garlic. Pour the stock over the tomatoes, moistening the rice thoroughly. Cover the dish and bake for 25 to 30 minutes or until the rice is tender, basting occasionally.

6. Garnish with chopped parsley, and serve immediately.

POWERFOOD HIGHLIGHT
Tomatoes, brown rice, pecans, garlic, parsley

Brown Rice with Burdock

Serves 8

*b*urdock, not your everyday root vegetable, is very popular in Japan. In this country it can be found in Asian markets and some health food stores. It grows wild in the colder parts of North America and the root is harvested in June and July. Most people are familiar with burdock via its nasty burrs that stick onto your dog and your clothes in the fall. For a subtle taste treat, I like to combine burdock with brown rice and perky veggies such as scallions and chives.

1 tablespoon canola oil
½ pound burdock root, peeled and shredded
2 teaspoons sea salt
2 cups long-grain brown rice
½ cup drained and diced canned pimientos
½ cup chopped scallions
¼ cup chopped chives

1. In a saucepan, heat the canola oil and add the burdock. Cook 3 minutes.

2. Add 4 cups cold water and the sea salt. Cover and bring to a boil.

3. Remove cover and add rice. Cover and cook until rice is cooked, about 45 minutes.

4. When rice is tender, add pimientos, chopped scallions, and chives and mix well.

POWERFOOD HIGHLIGHT
Burdock, brown rice, pimientos, scallions, chives

Buckwheat Noodles with
Spicy Peanut Sauce
Serves 8

*f*or you peanut lovers, here's a
simple but sophisticated way to enjoy your favorite snack food
in a healthy, protein-rich, and very flavorful recipe. This dish can
be enjoyed anytime of year, but it's especially good in the summer
months, as very little cooking is required. Add a green salad or
steamed vegetables to round out a meal.

¼ cup all natural peanut butter
1 cup chicken stock or vegetable stock
1 tablespoon tamari
2 tablespoons sugar
¼ teaspoon red pepper flakes
2 tablespoons dark sesame oil
8 ounces (1 package) buckwheat soba noodles
¼ cup chopped peanuts
1 tablespoon chopped fresh cilantro

1. In a medium bowl, whisk the peanut butter, stock, tamari,
sugar, red pepper flakes, and sesame oil.

2. Cook the soba noodles according to manufacturer's instructions.

3. After you have drained the noodles, toss them in a bowl with
the sauce.

4. Add chopped peanuts and fresh cilantro. Serve immediately.

POWERFOOD HIGHLIGHT
*Red pepper flakes, buckwheat soba noodles,
peanuts, cilantro*

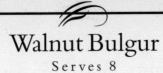

Walnut Bulgur
Serves 8

*t*he walnuts add a wonderful crunch to this whole-grain recipe and also provide additional protein and fiber. It's quick and easy to make, freezes well, and can be microwaved back to hot in minutes. It's a perfect base for a bok choy or broccoli stir-fry, and can also stand on its own, accompanied by a salad. I love this recipe not only for its great taste and texture, but also for its versatility.

1 quart chicken stock or vegetable stock, or water
2 cups bulgur wheat
2 tablespoons minced onion
1 stalk celery, minced
2 tablespoons chopped fresh basil
¼ cup chopped walnuts
½ tablespoon soy sauce
¼ cup chopped fresh parsley

1. In a large saucepan, bring the chicken stock to a boil over high heat.

2. Lower the temperature to a simmer; add the bulgur, onion, celery, and basil. Cover and cook for 5 minutes. Remove from the heat and set aside, covered, for 10 to 15 minutes.

3. Stir in walnuts, soy sauce, and chopped parsley. Serve at once.

POWERFOOD HIGHLIGHT
Bulgur wheat, onion, celery, basil, walnuts, parsley

Chapter 24

Entrées

*t*hese PowerFood entrées
are primarily comprised of grains and legumes, but
you will also find some non–PowerFoods here.
That's in keeping with the idea of balance, variety, and
moderation that should guide your eating. If pasta
is the entrée, the sauce will be a PowerFood sauce.
Or, where animal protein is at the center of the dish,
it will typically be fish, the healthiest of the animal
proteins. What's more, although we call these entrées,
they need not be taken in enormous portions
nor as the center of the meal. Combine them with
appetizers, soups, salads, or vegetable side dishes
for perfect PowerFood meals.

Basil Couscous with Squash
Serves 4

i prepare this recipe all summer with yellow summer squash and zucchini. In the fall and winter I switch to my all-time favorite—buttercup squash—which I serve with basil I have chopped and frozen from my summer crop, or fresh parsley, available year-round.

1 teaspoon extra virgin olive oil
¾ teaspoon salt
1 cup fresh basil leaves, cut in thin strips
½ cup couscous
2 cups squash in ¼-inch dice, steamed until tender

1. In a medium saucepan bring ¾ cup water to a boil.
2. Stir in the olive oil, salt, and basil. Boil until the basil is wilted.
3. Add the couscous and remove the pan from the heat. Let stand, covered, for 5 minutes.
4. Fluff the couscous with a fork, combine it with the steamed squash, and serve warm.

POWERFOOD HIGHLIGHT
Basil, couscous, squash

Barley Risotto
Serves 4

*b*arley is a healthy and delicious alternative to rice and pasta, and is a wonderful base for a wide variety of PowerFoods. This dish makes a substantial main course that needs only a green salad or side vegetable as accompaniment.

⅔ cup pearl barley
1 tablespoon extra virgin olive oil
1 chopped scallion
2 carrots, peeled and diced small
2 stalks celery, diced small
2 large leeks, thoroughly cleaned, white parts diced small
½ cup chicken stock or vegetable stock
½ cup grated Romano cheese
Handful of fresh parsley, chopped

1. Place the barley in a saucepan with 1½ cups water. Bring to a boil, lower the heat to a simmer, and cook until the barley is soft, about 40 to 50 minutes. Drain any excess water and set the barley aside.

2. In a large skillet, heat the olive oil over medium heat and sauté the scallion, carrots, celery, and leeks until tender. Pour the stock over the vegetables and cook over medium heat until the liquid is reduced by half. Stir the barley into the vegetables and cook until the barley is heated. Stir in the Romano cheese. Garnish with parsley and serve.

POWERFOOD HIGHLIGHT
Pearl barley, scallion, carrots, celery, leeks, parsley

Brown Rice Pilaf

Serves 4

*t*his very basic recipe is a wonder-ful convenience food. It freezes well and can always be available to accompany your favorite vegetable or fish recipes.

1 tablespoon canola oil
1 medium onion, finely diced
4 carrots, diced
4 stalks celery, diced
1¼ cups brown rice
2½ cups chicken stock or vegetable stock or water
1½ teaspoons chopped fresh thyme or ½ teaspoon
    dried thyme
1 tablespoon chopped fresh parsley
2 or 3 cloves garlic, peeled and finely chopped
Salt and freshly ground black pepper to taste

1. Preheat the oven to 350°F.

2. In a large saucepan, heat the oil and sauté the onion, carrots, and celery over low heat for about 8 minutes.

3. Add the rice and continue to cook until rice is lightly browned.

4. Remove from the heat, add the remaining ingredients, and mix well.

5. Transfer the mixture to a 1-quart casserole and bake, covered, for 30 to 40 minutes, until liquid is absorbed and rice is soft.

POWERFOOD HIGHLIGHT
Onion, carrots, celery, brown rice, thyme, parsley, garlic

Bulgur, Kale, and Carrot Pilaf

Serves 4

*b*ulgur is a flavorful and versatile whole grain. This recipe, which contains four different PowerFood groups, is as nutritious as it is quick and easy.

1 teaspoon canola oil
1 medium onion, coarsely chopped
3 cups chicken stock or vegetable stock
1 cup coarsely chopped fresh kale leaves
1 large carrot, diced
1½ cups bulgur
2 tablespoons freshly chopped chives
Salt and fresh ground black pepper to taste

1. Heat the oil in a large saucepan and sauté the onion in the oil over medium-high heat until just soft.

2. Stir in the stock, kale, carrot, and bulgur.

3. Bring to a boil and cook, covered, over low heat for about 10 minutes or until the liquid is absorbed.

4. Remove from the heat and stir in the chives. Season with salt and pepper.

POWERFOOD HIGHLIGHT
Onion, kale, carrot, bulgur, chives

Lentil and Brown Rice Casserole

Serves 8

*t*his dish is an ample main course, especially when topped with your favorite vegetables. I top it with a stir-fry of cauliflower, yellow squash, and red peppers. It keeps in the refrigerator for several days and freezes well.

1 cup brown rice
6 cups vegetable stock
2 cloves garlic, peeled and minced
1 tablespoon freshly chopped basil
2 tablespoons extra virgin olive oil
2 cups lentils
12 carrots, sliced into small angled chunks (rotate the
    carrot ¼ turn after each cut)
2 cups diced celery
1 small onion, diced
Salt and freshly ground black pepper to taste

1. Place the rice, vegetable stock, garlic, basil and olive oil in a large pot.

2. Rinse and pick over the lentils.

3. Add the lentils and vegetables to the pot. Bring to a boil, stir once, cover, reduce heat to a simmer, and cook for 45 minutes or until liquid is absorbed and vegetables are tender.

4. Season with salt and pepper to taste.

POWERFOOD HIGHLIGHT
Brown rice, garlic, basil, lentils, carrots, celery, onion

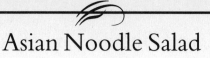

Asian Noodle Salad

Serves 4

I serve this spicy main dish for lunch and light dinners. Sometimes I add steamed chicken breasts, scallops, or even chopped walnuts or pecans for variety.

½ pound buckwheat soba noodles
1½ teaspoons canola oil
2 cloves garlic, peeled and minced
2 tablespoons coarsely chopped fresh ginger
1 teaspoon freshly squeezed lime juice
1 tablespoon soy sauce
2 tablespoons rice wine vinegar
1 teaspoon Chinese chili sauce
1 teaspoon chopped cilantro
1 teaspoon lemon zest
1 teaspoon red pepper flakes
½ cup blanched snow peas
2 carrots, julienned and blanched
1 cup mung bean sprouts

1. Cook the noodles according to package directions. Put the drained noodles in a large salad bowl and set aside.

2. In a sauté pan, heat the canola oil over medium heat and sauté the garlic and ginger until softened but not browned, approximately 2 to 3 minutes.

3. Add the lime juice, soy sauce, and rice vinegar. Simmer over medium heat for 1–2 minutes.

4. Add the Chinese chili sauce, cilantro, lemon zest, and red pepper flakes to the sauce. Pour the sauce over the noodles and toss well.

5. Combine the noodles with the snow peas, carrots, and bean sprouts, mixing well.

POWERFOOD HIGHLIGHT
Buckwheat soba noodles, garlic, ginger, lime juice, cilantro, lemon zest, red pepper flakes, snow peas, carrots, bean sprouts

Pasta with Papaya Salsa

Serves 4

*t*his unusual sauce is a refreshing break from tomato sauce. Its chunky texture nicely complements a flat pasta such as linguine or fettucine.

2 ripe papayas, peeled, seeded, and diced
2 or 3 poblano peppers, seeded and diced
½ medium red pepper, seeded and diced
2 tablespoons chopped fresh cilantro
Freshly squeezed juice of 1 lime
1 clove garlic, peeled and chopped
2 tablespoons extra virgin olive oil
1 pound pasta

1. In a mixing bowl combine all the ingredients except the pasta.
2. Cook the pasta according to package instructions.
3. In a large serving bowl, combine the drained pasta with the salsa and serve hot or warm.

POWERFOOD HIGHLIGHT
Papaya, peppers, cilantro, lime, garlic

Pasta with Quick Black Bean Sauce

Serves 4

*t*his sauce is a colorful combination of black and orange that is a snap to prepare on short notice. The sauce also makes an excellent topping for whole grains like brown rice, bulgur, and barley.

½ tablespoon extra virgin olive oil
1 carrot, diced
6 cloves garlic, peeled and minced
½ small onion, diced
2 cup cooked black beans (if using canned beans, rinse and drain)
3 scallions, chopped
1 tablespoon soy sauce
¾ pound pasta

1. In a saucepan, heat the olive oil over medium-high heat.
2. Sauté the carrot for 5 minutes. Add the garlic and onion and continue to cook until the vegetables are soft. Add the beans and cook for 5 more minutes.
3. Mix in the scallions and soy sauce.
4. Cook the pasta according to package instructions.
5. In a large serving bowl, toss the bean mixture with the pasta and serve immediately.

POWERFOOD HIGHLIGHT
Carrot, garlic, onion, black beans, scallions

Pasta with Zucchini Sauce

Serves 6 to 8

*t*his summer sauce is a favorite in July and August when the garden explodes with zucchini. I make it in large quantities and freeze the batches for use all year round. My favorite pasta for this sauce is rotini, especially four-color rotini. Other pasta that will hold sauce in its nooks and crannies are fusilli, shells, and even the plebian elbow macaroni.

1½ tablespoon extra virgin olive oil
3 cloves garlic, peeled and chopped
1 medium onion, chopped
4½ cups coarsely diced zucchini
1½ cups vegetable stock or chicken stock
Salt and freshly ground black pepper to taste
½ teaspoon chopped fresh basil
½ teaspoon chopped fresh oregano
1 pound pasta
1 ripe tomato, seeded and diced
6 tablespoons freshly grated Parmesan cheese

1. In a large skillet, heat the olive oil over medium heat.
2. Add the garlic, onion, and zucchini and sauté until tender.
3. Add the stock, salt, and pepper to the skillet and cook, uncovered, over medium heat for 5 minutes.
4. Remove the mixture from the skillet and purée in a blender with the basil and oregano.
5. Cook the pasta according to package directions.
6. Pour zucchini sauce over the pasta and scatter diced tomato and Parmesan cheese on top at serving time.

POWERFOOD HIGHLIGHT
Garlic, onion, zucchini, basil, oregano, tomato

Root Vegetables and Lamb Stew

Serves 6

*M*y version of lamb stew focuses on the vegetables and suggests a small quantity of lamb, whose rich flavor goes a long way. For a delicious taste treat, briefly sauté the turnips and carrots in a little butter, sprinkle with sugar, and caramelize before adding to the stew.

3 tablespoons canola oil

1½ pounds leg of lamb, well trimmed and cut into
    1-inch cubes

2 medium onions, diced

3 tablespoons flour

3 cups meat stock or water

6 medium potatoes, peeled and cubed

6 medium white turnips, peeled and cubed

6 medium carrots, sliced ½ inch thick

2 cloves garlic, peeled and minced

Salt and freshly ground black pepper to taste

2 tablespoons chopped fresh parsley

1. In a large skillet, heat the oil over medium heat. Add the lamb and brown on all sides. Remove the lamb from the skillet and set aside.

2. Add the diced onions to the same skillet and sauté briefly until they are translucent.

3. Place the lamb and onions in a large dutch oven. Sprinkle with the flour and mix well to coat the lamb and onions.

4. Add the stock or water and bring the stew to a boil. Stir from the bottom of the pan occasionally to prevent sticking.

5. Reduce the heat and simmer, covered, 1 hour. Skim the top with a ladle occasionally to remove any foam.

6. Add the potatoes, turnips, carrots and garlic. Continue to simmer for approximately ½ hour more, until the lamb and vegetables are tender.

7. Season with salt and pepper, and garnish with chopped parsley.

POWERFOOD HIGHLIGHT
Onions, turnips, carrots, garlic, parsley

Scrambled Tofu Fiesta

Serves 6

i call this dish a fiesta because it is light, colorful, and cheering. It is a flavorful way to introduce yourself to the health benefits of tofu. To save time, buy tofu that is sold already crumbled. Serve in a warmed whole grain burrito.

    2 tablespoons canola oil
    2 small onions, chopped
    1 red bell pepper, seeded and diced
    1 yellow bell pepper, seeded and diced
    1 tablespoon tamari
    ¼ teaspoon turmeric
    1½ pounds firm tofu, crumbled

1. In a medium skillet, heat the oil over medium heat. Sauté the onions and peppers until softened. Sprinkle with tamari and turmeric and mix well.

2. Add the tofu and mix, stirring constantly, until thoroughly heated.

3. Serve warm.

POWERFOOD HIGHLIGHT
Onions, peppers, turmeric, tofu

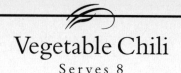

Vegetable Chili
Serves 8

*t*his faithful vegetarian standby is a cool weather favorite of mine. I serve it over brown rice, accompanied by a green salad.

1 tablespoon extra virgin olive oil
3 medium onions, diced
4 cloves garlic, peeled and diced
1 small green bell pepper, seeded and diced
1 jalapeño pepper, seeded and diced
1 stalk celery, diced
2 carrots, diced
1 small zucchini, diced
2 tomatoes, diced
1 tablespoon chili powder
1 tablespoon chopped fresh oregano or 1½ teaspoons dried
1 teaspoon cumin
2 (13½-ounce) cans red kidney beans, drained and rinsed
4 cups tomato juice

1. Heat the olive oil over low heat in a large saucepan. Sauté the onions, garlic, green pepper, jalapeño, celery, and carrots until the vegetables are tender, adding a small amount of water if necessary to prevent sticking.

2. Add the zucchini and tomatoes. Cook for another 2 minutes.

3. Add the remaining ingredients and mix thoroughly. Simmer, partially covered, over low heat for 35 minutes.

4. Serve hot.

POWERFOOD HIGHLIGHT
Onions, garlic, green pepper, jalapeño pepper, celery, carrots, zucchini, tomatoes, chili powder, oregano, cumin, red kidney beans, tomato juice

Vegetable Calzone
Serves 5

*t*his calzone is a substantial lunch or dinner. It takes some time to make the dough, but the results are worth it. Try it with Yellow Pepper Sauce (page 308).

Dough
½ tablespoon yeast
1 cup warm water
½ tablespoon extra virgin olive oil
1 cup all-purpose flour
1½ cups whole wheat flour
1 teaspoon celery salt

Filling
2 teaspoons extra virgin olive oil
2 red onions, cut into thin strips
2 unpeeled medium eggplants (approximately 6" long), diced
4 ripe tomatoes, diced
2 cloves garlic, peeled and minced
1 cup chopped fresh spinach
2 tablespoons chopped Spanish olives
¼ cup chopped fresh basil
2 tablespoons chopped fresh oregano
¼ cup soy nuts

1. In a large mixing bowl, dissolve the yeast in the warm water. When the water becomes frothy, stir in the olive oil. Slowly add the two kinds of flour, working them into the dough with a wooden spoon. Add the celery salt and mix it well.

2. Place the dough on a lightly floured surface and knead it for 2 to 3 minutes. Shape it into a ball, place it in a lightly oiled bowl, and cover with damp towel. Put the dough in a warm place and let it rise for 30 minutes.

3. Punch the dough down to deflate it, and divide it into 5 equal parts. On a lightly floured surface, roll the pieces into balls. With a rolling pin, roll each ball into a 6-inch circle.

4. Preheat the oven to 325°F.

PowerFoods

5. Heat the oil over medium heat in a large sauté pan. Sauté the red onions until translucent.

6. Add the eggplant and cook 10 minutes until the eggplant is softened, adding a small amount of water if necessary to prevent sticking.

7. Add the tomatoes, garlic, spinach, and olives. Sauté for 3 minutes. Add the basil, oregano, and soy nuts and cook for 1 minute more.

8. Place ¾ cup vegetable mixture on one side of each 6-inch circle of dough. Fold the dough in half and crimp the edges with a fork to be sure they are completely sealed. Place the calzones on a lightly greased baking sheet and bake for 15 minutes.

POWERFOOD HIGHLIGHT
Whole wheat flour, red onions, eggplant, tomatoes, garlic, spinach, olives, basil, oregano, soy nuts

Baked Halibut with Herb Bread Crumb Topping

Serves 4

*t*his fish entrée is delicious served with Citrus Asparagus Salad (page 223), Walnut Bulgur (page 272), or any other whole grain or vegetable accompaniment.

2 teaspoons canola oil
1 red pepper, seeded and finely chopped
2 scallions, white and green parts finely chopped
1 clove garlic, peeled and minced
¼ cup fine bread crumbs
1 teaspoon chopped chives
1 teaspoon chopped fresh parsley
4 (4-ounce) halibut fillets
¼ cup nonfat mayonnaise or yogurt
Salt and freshly ground black pepper to taste
Lemon wedges

1. In a large sauté pan, heat the oil over medium heat, and sauté the red pepper for 5 minutes. Add the scallions and garlic and continue to cook until soft.
2. Preheat the oven to 375°F.
3. Remove the pepper mixture from the heat and stir in the bread crumbs, chives, and parsley.
4. Spread the top of the halibut fillets with mayonnaise or yogurt. Sprinkle the fillets with the crumb topping and bake them for about 15 to 20 minutes or until the fish flakes easily with a fork. Season with salt and pepper and serve garnished with lemon wedges.

POWERFOOD HIGHLIGHT
Red pepper, scallion, garlic, chives, parsley, lemon

Baked Trout with Corn Salsa
Serves 8

*t*his light and zesty salsa is especially good with such oily fish as trout, bluefish, and pompano. The salsa keeps for a week in the refrigerator.

Corn Salsa
1 cup fresh or frozen thawed corn kernels
¼ green pepper, seeded and diced
½ red pepper, seeded and diced
½ medium onion, diced
⅔ cup freshly squeezed lemon juice
⅔ cup freshly squeezed lime juice
2 teaspoons seeded, diced chili pepper
6 sprigs fresh cilantro, finely chopped

---

8 (6-ounce) trout fillets

1. In a small nonreactive bowl, combine the corn, peppers, onions, lemon juice, lime juice, and chile pepper. Stir to mix the vegetables well.
2. Chill for at least 1 to 2 hours.
3. Broil trout fillets for 5 to 7 minutes or until they flake easily with a fork. Garnish with salsa and cilantro.

POWERFOOD HIGHLIGHT
Corn kernels, peppers, onion, lemon juice,
lime juice, cilantro

Grilled Salmon with Fruit Sauce
Serves 4

Salmon is a very popular fish for its health benefits and versatility. The sweet and spicy Asian sauce is low in fat and high in flavor.

Fruit Sauce
3 tablespoons rice wine vinegar
1 tablespoon dark sesame oil
2 tablespoons soy sauce
½ cup thawed pineapple juice concentrate
¼ teaspoon ground ginger
¼ teaspoon sugar
1 clove garlic, peeled and minced
1 tablespoon cornstarch

_____

4 (6-ounce) salmon fillets, skin and pin bones removed

1. Combine the rice wine vinegar, sesame oil, soy sauce, pineapple juice, ginger, sugar, and garlic in a saucepan and bring to a boil.

2. In a small cup, dissolve the cornstarch in 1 tablespoon water. Stir the cornstarch into the sauce mixture and continue boiling, stirring constantly, until the sauce thickens.

3. Broil the salmon fillets for 5 to 7 minutes or until they flake easily with a fork.

4. Pour the sauce over the fish and serve.

POWERFOOD HIGHLIGHT
Pineapple juice, ginger, garlic

Salmon Teriyaki
Serves 6

*t*his soy-based marinade is quick to prepare. The fruit juices in the teriyaki temper the saltiness of the soy.

Marinade
½ cup soy sauce
2 tablespoons rice wine vinegar
1 tablespoon freshly squeezed lime juice
1 tablespoon sesame oil
1 tablespoon minced fresh ginger
1½ cups defrosted apple juice concentrate
¼ cup chopped chives

_____

6 (6-ounce) salmon fillets

1. In a blender, combine the soy sauce, rice wine vinegar, lime juice, sesame oil, ginger, and apple juice concentrate. Blend until smooth.

2. Place salmon fillets in a glass baking dish and pour the teriyaki marinade over them. Sprinkle the fillets with chives and marinate in the refrigerator at least 1 hour or up to 8 hours.

3. Remove the salmon fillets from the marinade and grill them outdoors or bake in a preheated 350°F. oven for 10 to 15 minutes. Serve immediately.

POWERFOOD HIGHLIGHT
Lime juice, ginger, apple juice, chives

Grilled Tuna Steaks with
Ginger Mayonnaise
Serves 6

*t*una is delicious prepared in this spicy, colorful fashion. Other firm-fleshed fish steaks, like salmon, swordfish, and halibut, can be substituted if desired.

½ cup low-fat mayonnaise
2 tablespoons skim milk
1 tablespoon Dijon mustard
1 teaspoon minced fresh ginger
1 teaspoon freshly ground black pepper
1 ripe tomato, diced
1 tablespoon chopped chives
1 tablespoon chopped parsley
6 (6-ounce) tuna steaks

1. In a small bowl, whisk together the mayonnaise, skim milk, mustard, ginger, and black pepper. Mix in the tomato, chives, and parsley. Let stand at room temperature for 1 hour.

2. Grill the tuna steaks until they reach desired doneness and top with the ginger mayonnaise.

POWERFOOD HIGHLIGHT
Mustard, ginger, tomato, chives, parsley

Chapter 25

Sauces, Dressings, and Accompaniments

Sauces, dressings, and accompaniments are a marvelous way to introduce more PowerFoods into your diet without making drastic alterations in what you eat. For that reason, they make a good starting point for the PowerFoods novice. Instead of a radical departure in your eating plan, get an immediate boost in your PowerFoods intake just by dressing up your food—whether it's dips for enlivening crudités, sweet sauces for desserts, sandwich spreads, salad dressings, or elegant sauces for entrées. Whenever you wonder what you should "put on top of" a dish, here's the answer.

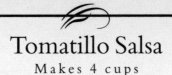

Tomatillo Salsa
Makes 4 cups

*V*ariety is the spice of life. If you've never had salsa made with tomatillos, you're in for a treat. After you've chopped, diced, and minced, the ingredients are easy to assemble, and the salsa keeps well in the refrigerator. I think the flavors actually blend and intensify more after a few days of storage. This salsa is great as a dip for toasted pita bread triangles, corn chips, or as a topping for potato, pasta or fish.

16 tomatillos, husked and diced
1 medium red onion, diced
4 jalapeño peppers, seeded and diced
4 cloves garlic, peeled and minced
¼ cup freshly squeezed lime juice
1 cup chopped cilantro
1 teaspoon sea salt

Place all the ingredients in a mixing bowl and stir well to combine thoroughly. Chill in the refrigerator for 2 to 4 hours before serving.

POWERFOOD HIGHLIGHT
Tomatillos, red onion, jalapeño peppers, garlic,
lime juice, cilantro

PowerFoods

Peanut Saté Dip
Makes ⅔ cup

*t*raditionally Thai in origin, peanut saté makes a delicious and unusual dip for grilled chicken cubes, steamed broccoli or cauliflower florets, chunks of carrot, blanched snow peas, or other vegetables of your choice. It's a quick and easy one-step way to dress up the crudités platter.

¼ cup vegetable stock
3 sprigs fresh cilantro, minced
2 tablespoons all natural peanut butter
2 tablespoons tamari
1 tablespoon rice vinegar
1 tablespoon honey
1 teaspoon dark sesame oil
½ teaspoon minced garlic
⅛ teaspoon red pepper flakes

1. Combine all the ingredients in a food processor and blend until smooth.
2. Transfer to a dipping bowl and chill.

POWERFOOD HIGHLIGHT
Cilantro, peanut butter, garlic, red pepper flakes

Warm Roquefort Dip

Makes 1½ cups

a dip to warm your inner depths and satisfy those cravings for comfort. Soy milk, parsley, shallot, horseradish, and walnuts stand up to the strength of Roquefort. I give this dreamy, creamy dairy and nondairy dip a five-star rating. For a party, serve it in a hollowed-out dark bread bowl surrounded by crudités.

1 (8 ounce) package nonfat cream cheese, softened
½ cup crumbled Roquefort cheese
3 tablespoons soy milk
1 tablespoon minced fresh parsley
1 shallot, minced
1 teaspoon grated horseradish
½ teaspoon tamari
¼ cup finely chopped walnuts

1. Preheat the oven to 350°F. degrees.
2. Place all the ingredients in a mixing bowl and stir to combine well.
3. Transfer the mixture to a small casserole dish. Bake for 15 to 20 minutes.
4. Serve warm.

POWERFOOD HIGHLIGHT
Soy milk, parsley, shallot, horseradish, walnuts

Cranberry Chutney

Makes 1 cup

*t*his tangy chutney can be served hot or cold. It is an ideal topping for whole grains and baked vegetables like onions and squash. It keeps well for up to one month in a covered container in the refrigerator.

1 cup fresh cranberries
¼ cup minced onion
¼ cup raisins
1 teaspoon freshly squeezed lemon juice
3 tablespoons defrosted apple juice concentrate
¼ teaspoon ground cloves
¼ teaspoon cinnamon
¼ teaspoon allspice

1. In a medium-size saucepan, bring the cranberries, onion, and ¼ cup water to a boil.

2. Reduce to a simmer, cover, and cook until tender, stirring frequently, about 35 to 40 minutes or until cranberries are soft.

3. Add the raisins and lemon juice. Cook 5 minutes longer, then add the remaining ingredients.

4. Divide the mixture in half.

5. Place one-half in a blender and blend until smooth. Mix the two parts together, put in a jar, and refrigerate.

POWERFOOD HIGHLIGHT
*Cranberries, onion, raisins, lemon juice, apple juice,
cloves, cinnamon, allspice*

Pineapple Apricot Chutney

Makes 2 cups

*C*hutney keeps up to one month in the refrigerator, and is therefore worth the little extra time required for its preparation. The unique combination of fresh and dried fruits is enhanced with the sweet tang of red onion and green Granny Smith apple. It is the perfect accompaniment to lamb or pork, or to serve on crackers for a quick appetizer. You may find that because this recipe is so deliciously savory, you're eating more chutney and less of everything else.

¼ cup sugar
½ ripe pineapple, peeled, cored, and cubed (about 1 cup)
½ cup cubed dried apricots
½ Granny Smith apple, skinned and cubed
1 small red onion, diced
½ cup raisins
1 tablespoon honey
1 teaspoon ground ginger
¼ teaspoon allspice
1 clove garlic, peeled and minced
1 cup apple juice

1. Place the sugar and 2 tablespoons water in a large saucepan and stir with a wooden spoon over medium high heat until the sugar is dissolved. Bring the mixture to a boil, stirring occasionally until a light brown syrup is achieved, about 3 to 4 minutes. Remove the syrup from the heat immediately.

2. Add the remaining ingredients and cook, covered, for 20 to 30 minutes over low heat.

3. Serve chilled or at room temperature.

POWERFOOD HIGHLIGHT
Pineapple, apricots, apple, red onion, raisins, ginger, allspice, garlic, apple juice

Mandarin Poppy Seed Dressing
Makes 1½ cups

*t*his basic salad dressing is a tangy, appealing way to incorporate tofu into your diet. It is delicious served on mesclun or your favorite greens.

½ cup soft tofu
2 tablespoons defrosted orange juice concentrate
¾ teaspoon dry mustard
2 tablespoons poppy seeds
1 tablespoon mayonnaise
¼ cup rice wine vinegar
¼ cup chopped shallots
12-ounce can mandarin orange sections, drained
Pinch of salt

Place all the ingredients in a blender and blend until smooth.

POWERFOOD HIGHLIGHT
Tofu, orange juice, mustard, poppy seeds, shallots, mandarin oranges

Miso Vinaigrette
Makes 1 cup

*L*oaded with PowerFoods, this Asian-flavored vinaigrette suits all kinds of raw greens as well as steamed broccoli florets and string beans.

2 tablespoons miso
2 tablespoons whole-grain mustard
¼ cup vegetable stock
2 tablespoons freshly squeezed lemon juice
2 tablespoons freshly squeezed lime juice
½ cup canola oil
2 teaspoons minced fresh ginger
1 scallion, minced
3 sprigs parsley, chopped
1 teaspoon chopped chives

1. In a mixing bowl, mix together the miso and mustard.
2. Whisk in the vegetable stock, lemon juice, and lime juice.
3. Add the oil in a slow, steady stream while whisking vigorously until the dressing is emulsified.
4. With a spatula, stir in the ginger, scallion, parsley, and chives.

POWERFOOD HIGHLIGHT
Miso, mustard, lemon juice, lime juice, ginger, scallion, parsley, chives

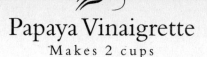

Papaya Vinaigrette

Makes 2 cups

*t*his vinaigrette inspires thoughts of a Caribbean holiday. It can serve as a marinade for swordfish, halibut, mahi-mahi, or other firm-fleshed fish. Chunks of chicken or pork also take well to these tropical flavors and when skewered into kabobs will make your grill sizzle. You can also thin the vinaigrette out and use it as a dressing for a salad of Bibb lettuce, chopped walnuts, and grapefruit sections.

4 very ripe papayas
1 teaspoon freshly squeezed lime juice
2 teaspoons defrosted orange juice concentrate
2 teaspoons defrosted pineapple juice concentrate
2 teaspoons red wine vinegar
1 teaspoon canola oil
Salt and freshly ground black pepper to taste

1. Peel and remove the seeds from the papayas. Place the flesh in a blender with the remaining ingredients and whip until smooth.
2. Add water if dressing needs to be thinned.

POWERFOOD HIGHLIGHT
Papaya, lime juice, orange juice, pineapple juice

Pineapple Mango Dressing

Makes 4 cups

*i*f you're not having your three fruits a day, here's a great way to get started. Fruits have not traditionally been used as dressings, but it's time to start a new trend. The concentrated full-bodied flavors of coconut and mango, together with the sweetness of pineapple, apple, and orange, are the inspiration we need. This versatile dressing can perk up a garden salad, grilled fish, or a dessert of sliced ripe fruit.

1 cup diced ripe pineapple
1 cup peeled and diced ripe mango
1 cup defrosted apple juice concentrate
1 cup defrosted orange juice concentrate
1 teaspoon sesame oil
¼ teaspoon coconut extract
¼ teaspoon salt

1. Purée all the ingredients in a processor or blender.
2. Chill and serve over baby greens or grilled fish.

POWERFOOD HIGHLIGHT
Pineapple, mango, apple juice, orange juice

Tofu Dill Mayonnaise

Makes 1¼ cups

*t*his recipe is a healthy substitute for regular mayonnaise, and nutritionally far superior to commercial low-fat or nonfat mayonnaise. It is a delicious and creative way to introduce tofu into your healthy eating plan. Use it liberally in any way that you would use mayonnaise.

1 box (10.5 ounces) silken tofu
¼ cup sherry vinegar
1 tablespoon Dijon mustard
2 teaspoons chopped dill

1. Combine all the ingredients in a blender and whip until smooth.
2. Place in a covered container and refrigerate for up to 4 days.

POWERFOOD HIGHLIGHT
Tofu, mustard, dill

Barbecue Sauce

Makes 3 cups

*t*his feisty sauce could not be more versatile. It is a great marinade for shrimp and chicken, a sauce for beef and lamb, and can be stirred into whole grains for lively flavor and powerful nutrients.

¾ cup defrosted orange juice concentrate

¾ cup chili sauce

⅓ cup molasses

3 tablespoons soy sauce

1 tablespoon brown mustard

2 cloves garlic, peeled and chopped

2 tablespoons freshly squeezed lemon juice

¼ cup chicken broth

1 teaspoon Tabasco sauce

2 tablespoons Worcestershire sauce

1. Combine all ingredients in a bowl and mix well.
2. Place the mixture in a saucepan and let it simmer, covered, for 15 to 20 minutes.
3. Adjust the seasonings according to your taste.

POWERFOOD HIGHLIGHT
Orange juice, chili sauce, molasses, mustard, garlic, lemon juice, Tabasco sauce

Fresh Tomato Sauce
Makes 4 cups

*t*omato sauce goes with nearly everything—pasta and grains as well as vegetables. Create your own variations by adding mushrooms, olives, more onions, or whatever you like.

2 tablespoons extra virgin olive oil
1 onion, finely chopped
3 celery ribs, finely chopped
2 carrots, diced
1 green pepper, seeded and finely chopped
3 garlic cloves, minced
12 large plum tomatoes, chopped
2 tablespoons finely chopped fresh basil leaves
1 tablespoon finely chopped fresh oregano
Salt and freshly ground black pepper to taste

1. In a large dutch oven or covered saucepan, heat the olive oil over medium heat. Add the onion, celery, carrots, green pepper, and garlic and sauté them approximately 10 minutes or until the vegetables begin to soften.

2. Add the tomatoes, basil, oregano, and salt and pepper to taste.

3. Simmer the sauce over low heat, covered, for about 1 hour or until it thickens to a chunky consistency.

POWERFOOD HIGHLIGHT
Onion, celery, carrots, green pepper, garlic, plum tomatoes, basil, oregano

Mushroom Marinara Sauce
Makes 6 cups

*t*his marinara sauce deserves to have "mushroom" as its first name. It is really chock full of mushrooms, and they put this basic zesty pasta topping in another league. For an earthier, more robust flavor, remember that the wilder cousins to the white mushroom, such as porcini, cremini, shiitake and portobello, are now available on your supermarket shelves.

½ cup chicken stock
1 medium onion chopped
4 cloves garlic, peeled and minced
1 tablespoon finely chopped fresh oregano
2 tablespoons finely chopped fresh basil leaves
2 bay leaves
2 cups sliced mushrooms
3 cups tomato sauce (canned or homemade)
2 cups tomato purée
Salt and freshly ground black pepper to taste

1. In a large saucepan, bring the stock to a boil over high heat. Reduce the heat to medium and add the onion, garlic, oregano, basil, and bay leaves. Simmer until the onions are tender.

2. Add the mushrooms and cook 5 minutes.

3. Add the tomato sauce, tomato purée, salt, and pepper. Cover and simmer approximately 1 hour over low heat. Remove the bay leaves before serving.

POWERFOOD HIGHLIGHT
Onion, garlic, oregano, basil, bay leaves, mushrooms, tomato sauce and purée

Mustard Chive Pasta Sauce

Makes 2 cups

*i*f you love mustard and are inter-
ested in exploring unconventional combinations, this recipe satisfies.
It's perfect for a pasta side dish or as a sauce for broiled or baked fish.

1 tablespoon extra virgin olive oil
1 medium onion, diced
6 tablespoons Dijon mustard
¼ cup prepared yellow mustard
½ cup chicken stock
1 tablespoon white wine
1 cup thin shreds of fresh spinach leaves
½ cup chopped chives
¼ cup half-and-half
1 large tomato, diced
Freshly ground black pepper to taste
¼ cup freshly grated Parmesan cheese

1. In a large sauté pan, heat the oil over medium heat and sauté
the onion until lightly browned
2. Stir in the mustards, stock, and wine and cook over medium
heat until the mixture is heated through, approximately 3 minutes.
3. Add the spinach, chives, half-and-half, tomato, and black
pepper. Mix well and once again heat thoroughly to just below the
boiling point.
4. Serve over pasta and sprinkle with Parmesan cheese.

POWERFOOD HIGHLIGHT
Onion, mustard, spinach, chives, tomato

Yellow Pepper Sauce

Makes 3 cups

*t*he mild flavor of yellow peppers spiced up with onion and Worcestershire sauce is great with pasta or fish. Experiment with orange or red peppers for a slightly stronger taste and burst of color.

2 cups diced yellow peppers
1 small onion, diced
1½ cups vegetable stock
1 teaspoon Worcestershire sauce
1 teaspoon chopped fresh basil
Salt and freshly ground black pepper to taste

1. In a saucepan, combine all the ingredients and bring to a boil. Lower the heat and simmer, covered, for 10 minutes.
2. Remove the mixture from the heat and place it in a blender. Purée until smooth.
3. Serve warm.

POWERFOOD HIGHLIGHT
Yellow peppers, onion, basil

Pesto
Makes 1 cup

*P*ungent, potent pesto depends on fresh basil for its classic Italian flavor. Make this in quantity in the summer when fresh basil is readily available. It freezes well, and so can be enjoyed year-round.

3 cups fresh basil leaves
¼ cup extra virgin olive oil
¼ cup water
2 tablespoons pine nuts
3 garlic cloves, peeled and roughly chopped
1 teaspoon salt
¼ cup freshly grated Parmesan cheese

1. Put the basil, olive oil, water, pine nuts, garlic, and salt in a blender or food processor and blend until smooth.
2. Stir in the Parmesan cheese.
3. Serve either warm or at room temperature.

POWERFOOD HIGHLIGHT
Basil, pine nuts, garlic

Blueberry Syrup

Makes 1½ cups

*t*his syrup is perfect in the morning served on pancakes and waffles, and for dessert spooned over angel food cake and fruit compote.

2 cups fresh or frozen blueberries
½ cup freshly squeezed orange juice
¼ teaspoon lemon zest
1 tablespoon chopped fresh mint
2 tablespoons sugar
½ teaspoon cinnamon
2 tablespoons cornstarch dissolved in ¼ cup water

1. Combine all the ingredients in a saucepan and bring to a boil. Reduce the heat to a simmer and cook, uncovered, stirring occasionally, until the sauce thickens to the consistency of maple syrup.
2. Serve warm.

POWERFOOD HIGHLIGHT
Blueberries, orange juice, lemon zest, mint, cinnamon

Orange Cherry Jubilee Sauce

Makes 1½ cups

a festival of flavors in a deliciously decadent, naturally fat-free sauce will bring a holiday air to your table. Delight your family and friends with this topping served over sliced ripe peaches or use it to power up your favorite frozen yogurt.

1 cup pitted bing cherries (canned in syrup and drained)
½ cup freshly squeezed orange juice
¼ cup brandy
2 tablespoon kirsch liqueur
2 tablespoons brown sugar
1 teaspoon cinnamon
1 tablespoon cornstarch
2 tablespoons water

1. In a saucepan, combine the cherries and orange juice over medium heat and bring to a simmer. Stir in the brandy and kirsch. Taking care to avert your face, set liqueurs aflame with a lighted match.

2. Continue to simmer until the flame burns out and then stir in the brown sugar and cinnamon.

3. In a separate bowl, combine the cornstarch and water and mix well.

4. Add the cornstarch mixture to the cherries, stirring constantly over medium heat until the mixture thickens, about 3 to 5 minutes. Serve warm.

POWERFOOD HIGHLIGHT
Bing cherries, orange juice, cinnamon

Raspberry Sauce
Makes 1½ cups

*i*ts name doesn't do justice to the intense burst of flavor in each spoonful of this sauce. Calling it "Sauce Framboise," thereby adding the French touch, might be more in keeping with its classic gourmet nature. Call it what you will, but do make it in raspberry season and freeze any extra for use later on. It is definitely a dessert recipe. Serve it over angel food or pound cake, frozen yogurt, or slices of fresh, ripe fruit.

2 cups fresh raspberries
½ cup sugar
⅓ cup framboise or other raspberry liqueur

1. In a blender or food processor, combine the raspberries, sugar, and liqueur. Blend until thick.

2. If desired, remove the raspberry seeds by pressing the sauce through a fine sieve into a bowl.

3. Refrigerate the smooth sauce until ready to use.

POWERFOOD HIGHLIGHT
Raspberries

Peach Butter

Makes 2 cups

*h*aven't you always wanted to make your own spread for bread but were afraid to try? This recipe is simplicity itself, and by using dried peaches you can make it all year-round. Peach butter is a concentrated PowerFood topping for hot cereals, breads, muffins, pancakes, and even the dieter's delight— rice cakes.

2 cups dried peaches
1 teaspoon ground cinnamon
½ teaspoon ground allspice
⅛ teaspoon ground cloves
2 cups apple juice
¼ cup granulated sugar
1 tablespoon freshly squeezed lemon juice

1. Combine all the ingredients in a large saucepan and bring to a boil over medium heat.

2. Reduce the heat to low. Cover and simmer for 20 minutes, stirring occasionally. Remove the sauce from the heat and let cool to room temperature.

3. Scrape into the bowl of a food processor and blend until smooth.

POWERFOOD HIGHLIGHT
*Peaches, cinammon, allspice, cloves, apple juice,
lemon juice*

Chapter 26

Breads, Muffins, and Pancakes

*e*verybody eats bread. It's the staff of life, even when it's in the form of muffins, and certainly when it's in the form of pancakes. The following breads, muffins, and pancakes do more than just satisfy the soul; they nourish the body. In addition to boring old flour and water, they have whole grains and, in many cases, vegetables and fruits, nuts and seeds. It means you can feel good about the breads you eat, not to mention the fact that they taste delicious.

Barry Bread
Makes 1 loaf

*C*hef Barry Correia's honey whole wheat bread is a basic, delicious, all-purpose recipe which can also be made into rolls or dressed with spices, nuts, and seeds. Cardamom, anise, and caraway are some of my favorite bread spices, and sunflower seeds are always welcome.

1 cup warm water
1 tablespoon yeast
1 cup all-purpose flour
3 cups whole wheat flour
2 eggs
4 teaspoons honey
2 tablespoons canola oil
Pinch salt

1. Combine the water and yeast in a large mixing bowl. Stir until the yeast dissolves.
2. In a separate bowl, combine the all-purpose flour and whole wheat flour. Mix well.
3. Add the eggs, honey, oil, and salt to the yeast mixture. Add the dry ingredients a little at a time, scraping the sides of the bowl, until all the flour is incorporated and the mixture forms a ball. If it seems too dry, add more water, 1 teaspoon at a time.
4. Knead a few times, just enough to shape the dough into a ball. Return the dough to the bowl.
5. Cover the bowl with a cloth and set it in a warm place to rise. Allow the dough to double in size (about 1 hour).
6. Spray a 9 × 5-inch loaf pan with nonstick vegetable spray.
7. Punch the dough down, remove it from the bowl, place it in the loaf pan, and allow it to rise again for approximately 1 hour or until doubled in size.
8. Heat the oven to 350°F.
9. Bake for 1 hour or until the loaf sounds hollow when tapped.

POWERFOOD HIGHLIGHT
Whole wheat flour, and spices, nuts and seeds if used

Corn Bread
Makes 9 squares

*W*ho doesn't enjoy corn bread? This moist and flavorful version with added vegetables is just about the best I've eaten. Enjoy it with all your whole grain and legume recipes, and by all means try it with Vegetable Chili (page 285). It's great for brunch, an informal buffet, and for any meal with a Southwestern theme.

1¼ cups stone-ground yellow cornmeal
1 cup all-purpose flour
⅓ cup sugar
1 tablespoon baking powder
¼ teaspoon baking soda
½ teaspoon salt
1 egg
1 cup buttermilk
¼ cup chopped green pepper
1 cup corn kernels
6 tablespoons canola oil

1. Preheat the oven to 400°F. Lightly grease a 9 × 9–inch cake pan.

2. In a large bowl, combine the cornmeal, flour, sugar, baking powder, baking soda, and salt.

3. In a small bowl, whisk the egg, then beat in the buttermilk. Add the buttermilk mixture to the dry mixture and stir until just combined.

4. Add the green pepper, corn, and canola oil and stir until the batter is thick and the solids well distributed.

5. Pour the batter into the cake pan. Bake for 30 to 35 minutes or until the top of the loaf is golden brown and springy to the touch.

POWERFOOD HIGHLIGHT
Yellow cornmeal, green pepper, corn kernels

Sweet Potato Gingerbread

Makes 1 loaf

*h*earty and substantial, this flavor-filled gingerbread has the added PowerFood benefit of sweet potato. This is truly a marriage made in heaven.

4 eggs
8 tablespoons honey
1½ cups cooked, mashed sweet potatoes
2 tablespoons molasses
2 teaspoons vanilla extract
2 cups all-purpose flour
2 teaspoons baking powder
2 teaspoons cinnamon
1 teaspoon ground ginger
½ teaspoon ground cloves

1. Preheat the oven to 375°F. Grease a 9 × 5-inch loaf pan.

2. In a large mixing bowl, beat the eggs for about 2 minutes.

3. Add the honey, sweet potatoes, molasses, and vanilla. Beat for 2 to 3 minutes until the mixture is smooth and uniform.

4. In a separate bowl, combine the flour, baking powder, cinnamon, ginger, and cloves.

5. Add the dry ingredients to the sweet potato mixture and stir until just mixed.

6. Scrape the batter into the loaf pan and bake for 20 to 30 minutes or until a toothpick inserted into the center comes out clean. Turn out on a rack to cool.

POWERFOOD HIGHLIGHT
Sweet potatoes, molasses, vanilla extract, cinnamon, ginger, cloves

Pumpkin Bread

Makes 1 loaf

*h*ere's a sweet pumpkin tea bread that is good any time of day topped with chutney or fruit spreads. For convenience, canned pumpkin is a highly acceptable and practical alternative to fresh-cooked pumpkin. You can also substitute sweet potato, yam, or winter squash purée in the same quantity as the pumpkin.

2 cups all-purpose flour
¼ teaspoon baking powder
1 teaspoon baking soda
1 teaspoon salt
½ teaspoon cinnamon
¼ teaspoon allspice
1 cup sugar
⅓ cup canola oil
3 eggs
1 cup canned or fresh cooked pumpkin purée
½ cup low-fat milk
¼ cup raisins

1. Preheat the oven to 350°F. Grease a 9 × 5-inch loaf pan.

2. In a large bowl, combine the flour, baking powder, baking soda, salt, cinnamon, and allspice.

3. In a separate large mixing bowl, combine the sugar, oil, and eggs and beat until fluffy. Add the pumpkin, milk, and raisins and stir to combine well.

4. Slowly add the dry ingredients to the pumpkin mixture and mix well.

5. Scrape the batter into the loaf pan and bake for approximately 1 hour or until a toothpick inserted into the center comes out clean. Loosen the sides and turn out on a rack to cool.

POWERFOOD HIGHLIGHT
Cinnamon, allspice, pumpkin, raisins

Banana Cherry Nut Bread

Makes 1 loaf

*t*his is banana bread with a difference, and that difference is the addition of dried cherries. The color specks and flavor of the cherries and the crunch of walnut bits make this bread special. If you make an extra loaf or two, slice before freezing for a quick "pick-me-up," one slice at a time.

1⅓ cups all purpose flour
1½ teaspoons baking powder
½ teaspoon baking soda
½ teaspoon salt
½ cup sugar
¾ cup (1½ sticks) butter, softened
2 eggs
⅓ cup skim milk
3 ripe bananas, mashed
¼ cup dried cherries
2 tablespoons chopped walnuts
1 tablespoon freshly squeezed lemon juice

1. Preheat the oven to 350°F.
2. Lightly grease the bottom only of a 9 × 5-inch loaf pan.
3. In a large mixing bowl, combine the flour, baking powder, baking soda, and salt and set aside.
4. In another large bowl, beat the sugar and butter until the mixture is light and fluffy. Add the eggs 1 at a time, beating well after each addition. Stir in the milk, beating until well mixed. Add the flour mixture, stirring it into the wet ingredients gradually, just until mixed.
5. Fold the mashed bananas, cherries, and walnuts into the batter.
6. Scrape the batter into the loaf pan and bake for 40 to 45 minutes or until a toothpick inserted into the center comes out dry.
7. Loosen the sides of the loaf with a knife and remove from the pan to a rack to cool.

POWERFOOD HIGHLIGHT
Bananas, dried cherries, walnuts, lemon juice

Bran Muffins
Makes 12 muffins

*W*heat bran, buttermilk and black-strap molasses add flavor and a good dose of power nutrients and fiber to the recipe. This is truly a bran muffin for "health nuts," and a tasty alternative to the high-fat bran muffins found in coffee shops, convenience stores, and supermarkets. Chopped nuts and/or dried fruits can be added to this easy muffin recipe for variety.

2 cups whole wheat flour
1½ cups wheat bran
2 tablespoons sugar
¼ teaspoon salt
1¼ teaspoons baking soda
2 cups buttermilk
1 egg, beaten
½ cup blackstrap molasses
2 tablespoons canola oil
1 cup raisins
2 tablespoons grated orange zest

1. Preheat the oven to 400°F. Grease 12 muffin cups.

2. Combine the wheat flour, wheat bran, sugar, salt, and baking soda in a mixing bowl and set it aside.

3. In a separate large mixing bowl, combine the buttermilk, egg, molasses, and oil just until mixed.

4. Gradually add the dry ingredients to the wet ones, stirring to combine them.

5. Fold the raisins and orange zest into the batter and divide the batter among the greased muffin cups.

6. Bake for 15 to 20 minutes or until a toothpick inserted into the center comes out clean.

POWERFOOD HIGHLIGHT
Whole wheat flour, bran, molasses, raisins, orange zest, and nuts and dried fruits (if used)

Buckwheat Muffins

Makes 12 muffins

*b*uckwheat flour is widely used for pancakes. Its hearty and rustic flavor, however, is not as familiar in muffins. Dates and molasses add a dark, delicious sweetness to the already aromatic buckwheat and help to achieve a moist and delicious treat. If you want to experiment, add extra liquid to the muffin ingredients to create a pancake batter consistency, so you can enjoy the more traditional use of buckwheat flour.

⅔ cup all-purpose flour

1⅓ cups buckwheat flour

1 teaspoon salt

2 teaspoons baking powder

¼ cup chopped dates

1 egg, beaten

2 tablespoons molasses

1 cup low-fat milk

1 teaspoon canola oil

1. Preheat the oven to 400°F. Grease 12 muffin cups.

2. Combine the all-purpose flour, buckwheat flour, salt, and baking powder in a bowl and set aside.

3. In a separate bowl, combine the dates, eggs, molasses, milk, and canola oil.

4. Add the dry ingredients to the egg mixture and mix to combine them well.

5. Spoon the batter into the muffin cups.

6. Bake the muffins for 20 to 25 minutes or until a toothpick inserted into the center comes out clean.

POWERFOOD HIGHLIGHT
Buckwheat flour, dates, molasses

Grape-Nuts Muffins
Makes 8 muffins

*b*reaking open this muffin is a treat for the senses. Imagine the aroma of the malted barley from the Grape-Nuts, the sight of the little jewels of tartly sweet dried cranberries, and the anticipated taste and crunch of golden walnut nuggets. This muffin has it all!

1 tablespoon canola oil

1 cup Grape-Nuts cereal

3 tablespoons honey

1 cup 1 percent milk

2 egg whites

¾ cup all-purpose flour

¾ cup whole wheat flour

1½ teaspoons baking powder

¼ teaspoon cinnamon

½ cup chopped walnuts

½ cup chopped dried cranberries

1. Preheat the oven to 350°F. Grease 8 muffin cups.

2. In a large skillet, heat the oil over medium heat and sauté the Grape-Nuts for 5 minutes until lightly toasted.

3. Add the honey and stir well to coat. Remove from the heat.

4. In a large bowl, beat together the milk, egg whites, and glazed Grape-Nuts until well mixed.

5. In a separate bowl, combine the all-purpose flour, whole wheat flour, baking powder, and cinnamon. Add to the Grape-Nuts mixture and mix well.

6. Stir the chopped walnuts and cranberries into the batter.

7. Fill the greased muffin cups ⅔ full of batter and bake the muffins for 20 minutes or until a toothpick inserted into the center comes out clean.

POWERFOOD HIGHLIGHT
Grape-Nuts, whole wheat flour, cinnamon,
walnuts, cranberries

Sweet Potato Muffins

Makes 12 muffins

*Y*ou can never have enough sweet potato in your life. If you love the convenience of muffins for breakfast, lunch, snack, or dessert, this recipe will become one of your favorites. The muffins freeze well and will also keep well-refrigerated for several days—if they don't get eaten first.

1¾ cups whole wheat flour
½ teaspoon salt
¼ cup brown sugar
2 teaspoons baking powder
1 teaspoon cinnamon
1 teaspoon nutmeg
2 eggs
2 tablespoons canola oil
¾ cup skim milk
1 cup cooked, mashed sweet potato
¼ cup chopped pecans

1. Preheat the oven to 400°F. Grease 12 muffin cups.

2. Combine the flour, salt, sugar, baking powder, cinnamon, and nutmeg in a mixing bowl.

3. In a separate large mixing bowl, combine the eggs, canola oil, skim milk, sweet potato, and pecans.

4. Slowly add the dry ingredients to the wet mixture, stirring until just mixed.

5. Spoon the batter into the muffin cups and bake 20 to 25 minutes or until a toothpick inserted into the center comes out clean.

POWERFOOD HIGHLIGHT
Whole wheat flour, cinnamon, nutmeg, sweet potato, pecans

Orange and Fig Muffins

Makes 12 muffins

*O*ats add a healthy dose of fiber and protein to this especially delicious fruit-filled muffin. Try one as an alternative to your morning bowl of oatmeal. Fresh figs are my favorite fruit. However, if necessary, you can substitute dried figs, as the recipe is too good to depend on the seasonal availability of fresh figs.

2 large fresh figs, peeled and finely chopped
1 cup plus 1 tablespoon all-purpose flour
1 cup regular oats
1 tablespoon baking powder
Pinch salt
2 teaspoons grated orange zest
1 teaspoon cinnamon
1 cup skim milk
2 egg whites, lightly beaten
⅛ cup honey
½ cup (1 stick) butter, melted

1. Preheat the oven to 450°F. Grease 12 muffin cups.

2. In a small bowl, toss the chopped figs in 1 tablespoon of the flour.

3. In a large bowl, mix the remaining flour, oats, baking powder, salt, orange zest, and cinnamon and stir to combine well.

4. In another large bowl, mix together the milk, egg whites, honey, and melted butter.

5. Gradually add the dry ingredients to the wet ones and fold in the figs.

6. Spoon the batter into the greased muffin cups and bake for 10 to 15 minutes or until a toothpick inserted into the center comes out clean.

POWERFOOD HIGHLIGHT
Figs, oats, orange zest, cinnamon

Sweet Potato Pancakes
Makes 15 to 18 (4-inch) pancakes

*t*his pancake batter is also delicious made in a waffle iron. The pancakes or waffles are sweet enough to be eaten unadorned, but I can't resist adding a drizzle (or torrent) of maple syrup. For variety, try topping them with Peach Butter (page 313).

2 cups cooked, mashed sweet potatoes
½ cup (1 stick) butter, melted
4 eggs
2 cups skim milk
1½ cups all purpose flour
1½ cups whole wheat flour
1 tablespoon baking powder
1 teaspoon salt

1. In a mixing bowl, combine the sweet potatoes, melted butter, eggs, and milk and blend until the mixture is smooth and uniform.

2. Add the flours, baking powder, and salt and stir to combine well. Let the batter stand for 15 minutes.

3. Preheat a griddle or skillet over medium-high heat.

4. For each pancake, ladle ¼ cup of batter onto the heated griddle and cook until golden brown. Flip the pancakes and cook the other sides until brown. Repeat until the batter is used, keeping the finished pancakes warm.

POWERFOOD HIGHLIGHT
Sweet potatoes, whole wheat flour

Rice Flour Pancakes

Makes 15 to 18 (4-inch) pancakes

*t*hese pancakes are very versatile. They can be topped with stir-fried vegetables for a lunch or dinner entrée; topped with fruit compote or purée for a healthy low-fat dessert; or eaten for breakfast in the more conventional pancake manner. In addition, rice flour is a good substitute for anyone who is allergic or sensitive to wheat.

> 2 cups rice flour
> 4½ teaspoons baking powder
> 2 teaspoons brown sugar
> 1 teaspoon salt
> 2 cups skim milk
> 1 egg, beaten
> 1 tablespoon canola oil
> Vegetable oil spray

1. In a large mixing bowl, combine all the ingredients and mix well.

2. Preheat a griddle or skillet and spray lightly with vegetable oil.

3. For each pancake, pour onto the hot griddle enough batter to form a 4-inch circle and cook pancakes until golden brown on one side. Flip the pancakes and cook the other sides until brown. Repeat until you've used all the batter, keeping the finished pancakes warm.

4. Serve warm.

POWERFOOD HIGHLIGHT
Rice flour

Chapter 27

Desserts

g o for it! What's life with-
out sweetness? And why should you have to worry
about fat and calories as you add sweetness? Here are
low-fat recipes that are also high in PowerFoods;
you'll do yourself good as you take in the gift of these
desserts. So splurge, but do go easy on the apricot
raisin bread pudding.

Apple Butter Cake

Serves 10

*t*he concentrated flavor of apple butter in this spiced loaf dotted with raisins and nuts is very satisfying. Other fruit butters, such as Peach Butter (page 313), can be substituted, but don't use anything as mild and liquid as applesauce. Enjoy a slice of this cake for afternoon tea with friends.

½ cup (1 stick) butter, softened
1½ cups sugar
1 whole egg, well beaten
2 egg whites
1 cup all-purpose flour
1 cup whole wheat flour
1 teaspoon baking powder
½ teaspoon baking soda
¼ teaspoon salt
1 teaspoon cinnamon
½ teaspoon nutmeg
½ teaspoon cloves
1¼ cups apple butter
½ cup raisins
2 tablespoons chopped pecans

1. Preheat the oven to 350°F. Grease and flour a 9 × 5 loaf pan.
2. In a large bowl, cream the butter and sugar until fluffy.
3. Add the egg and egg whites and beat well.
4. Combine the two flours with the baking powder, soda, salt, cinnamon, nutmeg, and cloves. To the butter and sugar, add the flour mixture alternately with the apple butter.
5. Stir in the raisins and pecans and mix thoroughly.
6. Scrape the batter into the pan. Bake for 1 hour or until a toothpick inserted into the center comes out clean. Remove from the pan and cool on a rack.

POWERFOOD HIGHLIGHT
Whole wheat flour, cinnamon, nutmeg, cloves, apple butter, raisins, pecans

Apple Cranberry Crisp

Serves 12

*a*fter you've finished peeling, coring, and slicing a dozen apples, this recipe is easy to assemble. It makes a dazzling and delicious holiday (or any day) dessert. Stock up on fresh cranberries when they're in season. They freeze well.

1 cup flour
1 cup sugar
1 egg
1 teaspoon baking powder
½ teaspoon cinnamon
3 tablespoons butter, melted
¼ cup chopped hazelnuts
12 apples, peeled, cored, and sliced
2 cups cranberries (fresh or frozen)

1. Preheat the oven to 375°F. Grease and flour a 13 × 9 × 2-inch baking dish.

2. In a large bowl, mix the flour, sugar, egg, baking powder, cinnamon, half of the butter, and chopped hazelnuts until it has a crumb texture.

3. Spread the apples and cranberries in the baking dish and drizzle the rest of butter over them. Sprinkle the crumb mixture on top of the fruit.

4. Bake for 35 to 40 minutes or until fruit is bubbly and the crisp topping is golden brown. Serve warm.

POWERFOOD HIGHLIGHT
Cinnamon, hazelnuts, apples, cranberries

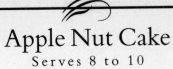

Apple Nut Cake

Serves 8 to 10

*t*his is a moist cake layered with sweet spiced apples and nuts. Its already delicious taste is heightened with the freshness of orange. If you want to keep fat grams to a minimum and flavor to a maximum, substitute applesauce for the oil.

4 large apples, cored, peeled, and sliced
2 tablespoons chopped walnuts
4 teaspoons cinnamon
2 cups sugar
3 cups flour
1 tablespoon baking powder
½ cup canola oil (or ½ cup applesauce for a
      low-fat alternative)
4 large eggs
½ cup freshly squeezed orange juice
1 tablespoon melted butter

1. Preheat the oven to 350°F. Grease a 10-inch angel cake pan or bundt pan.

2. In a medium bowl, blend the apples, walnuts, cinnamon, and ½ cup of the sugar.

3. In a separate bowl, combine the remaining 1½ cups sugar, the flour, baking powder, oil, eggs, orange juice, and butter. Beat 4 to 5 minutes to make a smooth batter.

4. Pour half the batter into the pan and spread half the apple mixture on top. Repeat the procedure and bake for 30 minutes. Then lower the oven temperature to 300°F. and bake 1 hour more or until a toothpick inserted into the center comes out clean.

POWERFOOD HIGHLIGHT
Apples, walnuts, cinnamon, orange juice

Baked Apples with Cherries and Walnuts

Serves 6

*e*asy is the operative word here. Easy to make, and even easier to eat. Try these cherry- and nut-filled baked apples for breakfast, brunch, or dessert.

2 tablespoons freshly squeezed lemon juice
⅓ cup dried cherries
3 tablespoons chopped walnuts
1 teaspoon grated lemon zest
2 tablespoons brown sugar
6 apples, cored

1. Preheat the oven to 375°F. Spray a baking sheet with nonstick vegetable spray.
2. In a bowl, mix together the lemon juice, cherries, walnuts, lemon zest, and brown sugar.
3. Place the cored apples on the baking sheet.
4. Fill each apple with 1½ tablespoons of the cherry-nut mixture.
5. Bake until the apples are soft, about 30 to 40 minutes.

POWERFOOD HIGHLIGHT
Lemon juice, cherries, walnuts, lemon zest, apples

Danish Applesauce
Makes 1 quart

*N*ot just your ordinary applesauce, this Danish version combines apples, citrus, and raisins into a zesty palate-pleaser. It's obviously perfect as is for dessert, makes a delicious crêpe filling, and can also serve as an accompaniment to poultry, game, or pork.

4 cups dried apples
¼ cup sugar
½ cup freshly squeezed orange juice
¼ cup freshly squeezed lemon juice
1 teaspoon allspice
1 cup raisins, soaked for 30 minutes in warm water

1. Place the dried apples in a saucepan and cover with water. Bring to a boil, reduce heat to a simmer, and cook, partially covered, for 15 to 20 minutes or until apples are plump and softened. Drain off cooking water.

2. Combine the apples, sugar, orange juice, lemon juice, and allspice in a blender. Blend to a chunky consistency.

3. Fold in the softened raisins.

POWERFOOD HIGHLIGHT
Apples, orange juice, lemon juice, allspice, raisins

Apricot Blackberry Cobbler

Serves 8

*A*pricots and blackberries are an unusual combination in an otherwise classic cobbler recipe. Fresh fruit is always my first choice, but I enjoy it just as much made with canned, drained apricots and frozen blackberries. Soy milk adds its own sweet, rich flavor but is not essential if it's not on hand. Substitute 1 percent or 2 percent milk in the same amount.

8 fresh ripe apricots, pitted and quartered
⅓ cup sugar
2 cups blackberries
1 cup plus 1 tablespoon all-purpose flour
½ cup whole wheat flour
¼ teaspoon salt
1½ tablespoons plus 1 teaspoon sugar
2 teaspoons baking powder
1 tablespoon grated orange zest
4 tablespoons (½ stick) butter, softened
¾ cup soy milk

1. Preheat the oven to 375°F. Grease an 8 × 8-inch baking dish.

2. In a small bowl, combine the apricots and ⅓ cup sugar. Set aside.

3. In a separate bowl, combine the blackberries and 1 tablespoon of the all-purpose flour. Set aside.

4. In a large bowl, combine the remaining all-purpose flour, whole wheat flour, salt, 1½ tablespoons sugar, baking powder, and orange zest.

5. Cut the butter into the dry ingredients until the texture is like a crumble and the dots of butter are the size of peas.

6. Add the soy milk, stirring just enough to moisten the dry ingredients.

7. Place the apricots and berries in the bottom of the baking dish and sprinkle the remaining 1 teaspoon of sugar over them.

8. Spoon the batter over the fruit and bake for 25 to 30 minutes or until the fruit is bubbly and the top is golden brown.

POWERFOOD HIGHLIGHT
Apricots, blackberries, whole wheat flour, orange zest, soy milk

Apricot Poppy Seed Cake

Serves 12

A melt-in-your-mouth cake, soft and creamy yet jazzed up just enough with poppy seeds and the flavor of rum to hold your interest. For me, the wonderful, healthy, delicious apricots are the prize.

2¼ cups all-purpose flour
1 teaspoon baking powder
¾ cup diced dried apricots
½ teaspoon salt
¼ cup (½ stick) butter, softened
⅔ cup sugar
1½ cups low-fat sour cream
3 egg whites, beaten until foamy
3 tablespoons poppy seeds
¼ teaspoon rum extract
Powdered sugar for garnish

1. Preheat the oven to 350°F. Lightly spray a bundt pan with nonstick vegetable spray.

2. In a bowl, mix together the flour, baking powder, dried apricots, and salt.

3. In a large bowl, cream the butter and sugar until light and fluffy. Beat in the sour cream and egg whites. Slowly add the flour mixture to the wet ingredients and mix just until thoroughly combined. Stir in the poppy seeds and rum extract.

4. Pour the batter into the pan and bake for 45 to 50 minutes or until a toothpick inserted into the center of the cake comes out clean. Let the cake cool on a rack for 10 minutes.

5. Loosen the cake from the sides of the pan with a knife. Remove the cake from the pan and let it cool on a rack. Sprinkle the cake with powdered sugar. Serve at room temperature.

POWERFOOD HIGHLIGHT
Apricots, poppy seeds

Baked Quince

Serves 4

*I*f you know someone with a quince tree in her backyard, you're in luck. Otherwise ask your produce manager to find some for you. Quince have a wonderful and unique flavor and this recipe brings out the best in them. You can combine several different chopped nuts (for example, almonds, walnuts, hazelnuts, pistachios) to vary the flavor.

4 large quince
½ cup unflavored bread crumbs
¼ cup chopped nuts
¼ cup brown sugar
1 tablespoon blackstrap molasses
2 tablespoons grated orange zest
2 tablespoons orange liqueur

1. Preheat the oven to 350°F.
2. Place the quince on a baking sheet and bake them for about 45 minutes or until almost tender.
3. Remove the quince from the oven (leave the oven on), and when they are cool enough to handle, core and hollow out about half of each fruit, placing the pulp in a mixing bowl.
4. To the quince pulp, add the bread crumbs, nuts, brown sugar, molasses, orange zest, and orange liqueur. Mix well.
5. Fill each quince shell with one-fourth of the mixture. Bake the quince for 15 minutes or until tender.
6. Serve hot or cold.

POWERFOOD HIGHLIGHT
Quince, nuts, molasses, orange zest

Fresh Strawberries Chantilly

Serves 8

Strawberries and cream! Need I say more? Well, I'll just mention something about fromage blanc. It's a lower-fat alternative to crème fraîche or whipped cream and is now available in the dairy section of many supermarkets. The strawberries, ideally, are ripe, juicy and bursting with flavor—perhaps just picked and purchased at your local farm stand.

8 cups fresh strawberries, washed, dried, hulled, and quartered
¼ cup brown sugar
¼ cup Grand Marnier or other orange-flavored liqueur
1½ cups fromage blanc or crème fraîche
8 mint sprigs

1. Place the strawberries in 8 attractive serving bowls.
2. In a mixing bowl combine the brown sugar, Grand Marnier, and either fromage blanc or crème fraîche, and mix well.
3. Place 3 tablespoons of the creamy mixture on top of each serving of strawberries and garnish all with a mint sprig.

POWERFOOD HIGHLIGHT
Strawberries, mint

Gingered Tangerines with Mint

Serves 6

*Y*ou can tango with these tangerines poached with ginger and red chile peppers. This is a combination that must be experienced; just reading the recipe won't reveal its true potential. It's light and refreshing and a perfect finish to a full-bodied meal.

  1 cup sugar
  1 dried red chile pepper, seeded and cut into strips
  2 cinnamon sticks
  ⅛ cup sliced fresh ginger
  6 tangerines, peeled and strings removed
  1 teaspoon freshly squeezed lime juice
  1 teaspoon freshly squeezed lemon juice
  1 teaspoon white vinegar
  6 large mint leaves, cut into strips
  ½ cup berries of your choice as garnish

1. In a saucepan, combine 6 cups of water, the sugar, chile pepper, cinnamon sticks, and ginger. Bring to a boil, then turn down the heat and simmer for 30 minutes, partially covered.

2. Add the tangerines and cook, covered, for 10 minutes, turning once to ensure even cooking. When done, remove the tangerines from the liquid and transfer them to a bowl. Put the poaching liquid back on the heat and simmer until it is reduced by ⅔. You should have about 1½ cups of liquid.

3. Remove the poaching liquid from the heat and stir in the lime juice, lemon juice, vinegar, and mint. Remove the cinnamon sticks. Pour the syrup over the tangerines and chill them overnight.

4. Serve the tangerines, mint, and syrup garnished with fresh berries.

POWERFOOD HIGHLIGHT
Red chile pepper, cinnamon, ginger, tangerines, lime juice, lemon juice, mint, berries

Dried Fruit Turnover

Makes 6 turnovers

a potpourri of simmered fruit and spices. Just delicious!

1 tablespoon butter
6 ounces dried fruits (apricots, raisins, cherries, and others)
3 tablespoons maple syrup
1 tablespoon freshly squeezed lime juice
1 teaspoon grated orange zest
½ teaspoon grated lime zest
½ teaspoon cinnamon
¼ teaspoon nutmeg
⅛ teaspoon ginger
24 sheets phyllo dough
1 egg white

1. In a saucepan, melt the butter and cook the fruit in it over moderate heat for 5 minutes.

2. Add ⅓ cup water, the syrup, lime juice, zests, and spices. Lower the heat and simmer the mixture until it is almost dry.

3. Spread out 6 phyllo sheets on the table and spray each one with nonstick vegetable spray. Add another layer of phyllo sheets and spray again. Continue adding phyllo and spraying each layer until there are 6 stacks, each with 4 phyllo sheets.

4. Fold the sheets in thirds lengthwise to form long rectangles.

5. Preheat the oven to 425°F.

6. Place one tablespoon of fruit mixture on one end of each rectangle, about 1 inch from the edge.

7. Fold the phyllo corner over the fruit into a triangle. Keep folding into triangles until done, like folding a flag.

8. Slightly beat the egg white with 1 teaspoon water, and brush the tops of the turnovers.

9. Bake 10 to 12 minutes until brown.

POWERFOOD HIGHLIGHT
Dried fruits, lime juice, orange zest, lime zest, cinnamon, nutmeg, ginger

Tropical Fruit Cup
Serves 4

*i*f you close your eyes as you sample the pineapple and coconut tastes, you may see palm trees swaying and ocean waves rolling onto the white sands of a tropical paradise. For a real fiesta, top this fruit cup with Cantaloupe Sorbet (page 344).

> 4 cups orange sections, free of seeds and membranes
> 2 cups peeled and diced fresh pineapple
> ¼ cup shredded coconut
> 2 tablespoons minced fresh ginger
> 2 tablespoons freshly grated orange zest
> 1½ cups orange juice
> ½ cup Cointreau or Grand Marnier

1. In a large bowl, combine the orange sections, pineapple, coconut, ginger, and orange zest. Toss very gently so the orange sections stay whole.

2. Pour the orange juice and liqueur over the fruit and chill overnight.

3. Remove the fruit with a slotted spoon to pretty cups and pour on as much juice as desired.

POWERFOOD HIGHLIGHT
Orange sections, pineapple, coconut, ginger, orange zest, orange juice

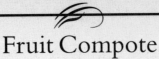

Fruit Compote
Serves 6

*g*reat for dessert, as a snack, or even an eye-opener at breakfast, this compote is a PowerFood powerhouse. Apple cider adds depth to this very simple dish. Don't confuse apple cider with its cousin apple juice, which is usually clear and strained free of solids.

1 cup dried cherries
1 cup dried apricots
1 cup diced dried figs
1 cup raisins
1 teaspoon cinnamon
¼ teaspoon ground cloves
2 cups apple cider

1. In a large saucepan, mix all the ingredients together and simmer for 1 hour.
2. Serve in bowls, warm or chilled.

POWERFOOD HIGHLIGHT
Cherries, apricots, figs, raisins, cinnamon, cloves, apple cider

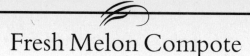

Fresh Melon Compote

Serves 4

*S*ummer heat calls for a cooling, refreshing dessert such as this. Look for really ripe, luscious melons to bring out the best in this recipe. For variety, try other melons such as casaba or Crenshaw.

2 cups watermelon balls or cubes
2 cups cantaloupe balls or cubes
2 cups honeydew balls or cubes
¼ cup sugar
1 cup sherry (nonalcoholic wine may be substituted)
1 cinnamon stick
Juice and grated zest from 1 lemon
4 mint sprigs (optional)

1. Put the melons, sugar, sherry, lemon juice, and zest in an attractive bowl.

2. Toss the fruit gently until the sugar is dissolved, about 1 to 2 minutes.

3. Add the cinnamon stick and chill for at least 2 hours.

4. Garnish with fresh mint if you like.

POWERFOOD HIGHLIGHT
Watermelon, cantaloupe, honeydew, cinnamon, lemon juice and zest, mint

Cantaloupe Sorbet
Makes 2 cups

*t*he addition of Pernod and lemon zest take this sorbet above and beyond anything you can buy. It's refreshing between courses or as a dessert, and well worth the effort involved.

½ cup sugar
2 tablespoons Pernod (optional)
2 (2-inch) strips lemon zest
1 tablespoon freshly squeezed lemon juice
3 ripe cantaloupes peeled, seeded, and coarsely chopped

1. In a saucepan, mix together ½ cup water, the sugar, Pernod, and zest.

2. Bring to a boil, stirring the mixture occasionally. Reduce the heat and simmer, uncovered, until the sugar is dissolved, about 5 minutes.

3. Stir in the lemon juice. Transfer the mixture to a large bowl and chill.

4. Blend the cantaloupe chunks in a blender or food processor until smooth, using a little of the syrup if needed to achieve a smooth consistency.

5. Mix the melon purée with the syrup until thoroughly combined. Strain the mixture through a sieve, pressing hard on the fibers that remain.

6. Place in an ice cream machine and freeze according to the manufacturer's directions.

POWERFOOD HIGHLIGHT
Lemon zest, lemon juice, cantaloupe

PowerFoods

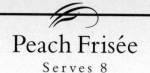

Peach Frisée

Serves 8

a cross between a smoothie and a pudding, this chilled brandy-spiked peach purée will dress up your favorite crystal. Top with berries and slivered almonds and you've got a dessert fit for royalty, or even your fussy family.

5 cups peeled sliced ripe peaches
1 tablespoon potato starch
¾ cup sugar
¼ cup brandy
½ cup fromage blanc or crème fraîche
½ cup fresh raspberries
¼ cup slivered almonds

1. In a saucepan, combine the peaches with 1¼ cups water and bring to a boil. Reduce the heat and simmer for 10 minutes. Drain.

2. Place the peaches in a blender and purée. Return them to the saucepan.

3. In a small bowl, dissolve the potato starch in 1 tablespoon water. Add it to the peaches and cook over medium heat for 5 minutes.

4. Remove the peaches from the heat and stir in the sugar and brandy.

5. Divide the peach purée among stemmed glasses and chill.

6. Top with fromage blanc or crème fraîche, raspberries, and slivered almonds. Serve cold.

POWERFOOD HIGHLIGHT
Peaches, raspberries, almonds

Pineapple Banana Shake
Serves 4

*b*ring out your best goblets, buy some tiny paper umbrellas, and dress up this shake for a luau any time of year. If you would like to serve this as a refreshing party punch, just add more Perrier or juice.

- 2 tablespoons grenadine
- 2 cups pineapple sorbet
- 1 tablespoon toasted coconut
- 2 bananas
- 1 teaspoon freshly grated lime zest
- 2 cups Perrier
- 1 cup pineapple juice

Combine all the ingredients in a blender and purée for 2 minutes. Serve over ice.

POWERFOOD HIGHLIGHT
Pineapple sorbet and juice, coconut, bananas, lime zest

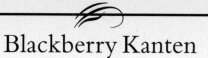

Blackberry Kanten

Serves 6

*S*ea vegetables for dessert? Well, yes. Agar-agar is a classic jelling agent from the sea. When it is combined with berries, it creates a healthy alternative to commercial, artificially colored and flavored gelatin desserts. The color and flavor of blackberries makes them my first choice, but for variety you can successfully substitute raspberries, blueberries, or small pieces of other fruits.

1 pint fresh blackberries
2 cups water
2 cups apple juice
⅛ teaspoon cinnamon
¼ cup sugar
⅛ teaspoon sea salt
¼ cup agar-agar flakes

1. Wash the blackberries and place them in a large saucepan.
2. Cover the berries with the water and the apple juice.
3. Bring the mixture to a boil and add cinnamon, sugar, sea salt, and agar-agar.
4. Cook at a simmer, uncovered, until thickened, approximately 10 minutes.
5. Pour the kanten into a dessert dish and let it chill in the refrigerator until firm.
6. Serve chilled.

POWERFOOD HIGHLIGHT
Blackberries, apple juice, cinnamon, agar-agar

Wild Blueberry Loaf

Makes 1 loaf

*t*ry this recipe with fresh wild blueberries if available. If not, make the effort to find frozen wild blueberries. These wild berries pack so much flavor in a tiny package that their taste will be your reward. A variation would be to substitute orange or pineapple juice for the milk.

¾ cup sugar

¼ cup (½ stick) butter, softened

1 egg

½ cup skim milk

2 cups flour

2 teaspoons baking powder

½ teaspoon salt

2 cups blueberries, washed and cleaned

Topping

⅓ cup sugar

⅓ cup flour

⅓ cup crushed gingersnaps

½ teaspoon cinnamon

2 tablespoons butter, softened

1. Preheat the oven to 350°F.

2. Mix together the sugar, butter, and egg. Stir in the milk. Add the dry ingredients.

3. Fold in the blueberries and place batter in greased 9 × 5-inch loaf pan.

4. Mix topping ingredients and sprinkle on top. Bake 45 to 50 minutes or until done.

POWERFOOD HIGHLIGHT
Blueberries, fruit juice if used, cinnamon

Apricot Raisin Bread Pudding

Serves 8

"Oh no," said the editor. "This recipe is just too rich to be part of our PowerFoods book." "Oh no," said I. "It's fabulous, it's my favorite, and we must have it." As you know, this book is not about deprivation. We all need such a dreamy, creamy dessert now and then. So indulge in a small portion for a special treat.

1 cup quartered dried apricots
2 tablespoons raisins
¼ cup (½ stick) butter at room temperature
12 thin slices Italian bread
Grated rind of 1 lemon
⅓ cup sugar
½ teaspoon cinnamon
Dash nutmeg
4 whole eggs
2 cups light cream

1. Preheat the oven to 350°F. Grease a 2-quart baking dish.

2. Cover the apricots and raisins with boiling water and let them stand for 5 minutes until they become plump. Drain the fruit and set aside.

3. Butter each slice of bread on one side and lay half the slices, buttered side up, in the baking dish.

4. Sprinkle the bread slices with half the apricots, raisins, lemon zest, sugar, cinnamon and nutmeg. Repeat steps 3 and 4.

5. Beat the eggs with the cream and pour the mixture over the bread and fruit.

6. Place the baking dish in a pan of water so that the water comes 1 inch up the sides of the baking dish. Bake for 1 hour or until the custard sets and the top is golden brown. Serve warm.

POWERFOOD HIGHLIGHT
Apricots, raisins, lemon zest, cinnamon, nutmeg

Basmati Rice Pudding

Serves 8 to 10

*b*asmati rice and apple juice add an aromatic flair to this low-fat version of the more traditional creamy rice pudding.

3 cups white basmati rice
2 cups apple juice
⅛ teaspoon sea salt
⅛ teaspoon cinnamon
⅛ teaspoon vanilla extract
½ cup raisins, soaked for 15 minutes in ¾ cup warm water

1. Preheat the oven to 350°F.
2. Place all the ingredients in a saucepan, cover, and cook over medium heat for 30 to 40 minutes or until the rice is tender.
3. Spoon the pudding into custard dishes and place in a water bath.
4. Bake for 20 to 30 minutes or until liquid is absorbed.

POWERFOOD HIGHLIGHT
Basmati rice, apple juice, cinnamon, vanilla extract, raisins

Papaya Fig Bruschetta

Serves 4

*b*ruschetta is traditionally served with tomatoes and garlic as an appetizer. My sweet variation makes a wonderful, unexpected treat for breakfast or dessert.

12 slices (½ inch thick) French bread
1 tablespoon melted butter
1½ tablespoons sugar
1 teaspoon ground cinnamon
1 fresh papaya, peeled, seeded, and finely diced
2 fresh figs, finely diced (see Note)
4 teaspoons low-fat plain yogurt
1 tablespoon honey

1. Preheat the oven to 375°F.

2. Lay the slices of bread on a baking sheet. Brush one side of each slice with butter and bake until golden, about 5 minutes.

3. In a small bowl, mix together 1 tablespoon of the sugar and the cinnamon. Sprinkle the mixture evenly over the buttered side of each slice of bread. Place the spiced toast under the broiler for 30 seconds. Remove and let cool.

4. In a bowl, stir together the papaya, figs, and remaining ½ tablespoon sugar. Place 1 tablespoon of the fruit mixture on each slice of bread. Top each slice with 1 teaspoon of yogurt and ¼ tablespoon of honey.

Note: Fresh figs have a very short season in the late summer. If they are unavailable, simmer dried figs in water or fruit juice for 10 minutes, remove from the heat, and let them soak for 10 minutes to reconstitute them.

POWERFOOD HIGHLIGHT
Cinnamon, papaya, figs

Whole Wheat Crêpes with Blueberry Filling

Makes 10 filled crêpes

*C*rêpes are always impressive and make a hit as a special dessert. These hearty, whole wheat crêpes and the blueberry filling can be prepared in advance and assembled at the last minute. A dollop of crème fraîche and/or a sprinkle of chopped nuts will add a gourmet touch. Make extra crêpes; they freeze well and can be filled with your choice of fruit spreads and served for breakfast or snacks.

Whole Wheat Crêpes
1½ cups whole wheat flour
2 cups evaporated skim milk
1 tablespoon sugar
3 tablespoons canola oil
4 egg whites, whipped until soft peaks form
2 teaspoons baking powder
1 teaspoon vanilla extract

1. Combine all the crêpe ingredients in a large bowl and mix until smooth. Let the batter rest for 10 minutes.

2. Preheat a nonstick crêpe pan or skillet over medium heat. Just before cooking, remove the pan from the heat and spray it with nonstick vegetable spray.

3. Add 2 tablespoons of batter, turning the pan from side to side to coat the bottom with a thin layer.

4. Return the pan to the heat and cook until the edges start to brown (2 to 3 minutes.)

5. Flip the crêpe and brown the other side. Repeat with the rest of the batter.

6. Place the prepared crêpes on a tray covered with a dampened towel in the oven on very low heat to keep warm.

7. Prepare Blueberry Filling (recipe follows).

Blueberry Filling
1 tablespoon cornstarch
1 tablespoon water
2 cups fresh blueberries
½ cup orange juice

1. Dissolve the cornstarch with the tablespoon of water in a small bowl. Set aside.

2. Place the blueberries and orange juice in a saucepan and bring to a boil.

3. Add the cornstarch to the berries, stirring constantly over medium heat. Cook until the mixture thickens to the consistency of a pie filling.

4. Place 2 tablespoons of warm filling on each crêpe and roll.

POWERFOOD HIGHLIGHT
Whole wheat flour, vanilla extract, blueberries, orange juice

Tofu Brownies
Serves 12

*t*ofu adds moisture and creamy consistency and acts as a replacement for fat. Tofu also adds the health benefits of soy to America's favorite treat. Eat these brownies without guilt. Now that's a twist.

1¼ cups cake flour
¾ teaspoon baking soda
½ teaspoon cinnamon
1 (10.5-ounce) package silken tofu
½ cup drained, puréed canned apricots
1 teaspoon canola oil
¾ cup sugar
¾ teaspoon almond extract
½ teaspoon pure vanilla extract
½ cup dry cocoa powder
2 tablespoons chopped pecans

1. Preheat the oven to 375°F.
2. Spray the sides of an 8 × 8-inch pan with nonstick vegetable cooking spray. Fit a square of waxed paper into the bottom of the pan and spray the top of the paper with cooking spray.
3. Combine the cake flour, baking soda, and cinnamon in a small bowl and set aside.
4. Place the tofu, apricots, oil, sugar, and almond and vanilla extracts in a blender and blend until smooth. Add the cocoa powder to the blender and blend 1 minute more.
5. Pour the mixture into a separate bowl and gradually mix in the dry ingredients. Blend well by hand with a wooden spoon.
6. Spread the batter evenly in the baking pan and sprinkle with chopped pecans.
7. Bake 20 minutes or until the center is set but remains moist. Do not overcook. Let cool in the pan on a rack before cutting into 12 portions.

POWERFOOD HIGHLIGHT
*Cinnamon, tofu, apricots, almond extract,
vanilla extract, pecans*

Chocolate Fondue Dip

Makes 2¾ cups

*f*ondue is fun. Chocolate is sublime, and dipping a favorite fruit PowerFood is perfection. End of story.

    12 ounces semisweet chocolate
    1 cup condensed low-fat milk
    1 teaspoon vanilla extract
    1 teaspoon brandy
    ½ cup skim milk
    Assorted cubed fruit

1. In a double boiler, combine the chocolate, condensed low-fat milk, vanilla, and brandy. Simmer.

2. When the chocolate is melted, add the skim milk, a tablespoon at a time, to thin to a dipping consistency

3. Keep the fondue warm in a chafing dish. Serve with cubed fruit for dipping.

POWERFOOD HIGHLIGHT
Vanilla extract, fruit

Further Reading

Barnard, Neal. *Food for Life.* New York: Crown Trade Paperbacks, 1993.

Brandt, Johanna. *The Grape Cure.* New York: A Beneficial Book, 1928.

Carper, Jean. *The Food Pharmacy.* New York: Bantam Books, 1988.
———. *Stop Aging Now!* New York: HarperCollins, 1995.

Colbin, Annemarie. *Food and Healing.* New York: Ballantine Books, 1986.

Goulart, Frances Sheridan. *Super Healing Foods.* West Nyack, NY: Parker Publishing Company, 1995.

Haas, Robert. *Eat Smart, Think Smart.* New York: HarperCollins, 1994.

Hausman, Patricia, and Judith Benn Hurley. *The Healing Foods.* New York: Dell Publishing, 1989.

Heinerman, John. *Heinerman's Encyclopedia of Fruits, Vegetables, and Herbs.* West Nyack, NY: Parker Publishing Company, 1988.

Katahn, Martin. *The Tri-Color Diet: A Miracle Breakthrough in Diet and Nutrition for a Longer, Healthier Life.* New York: Norton, 1996.

Lu, Henry C. *Chinese Foods for Longevity.* New York: Sterling Publishing Co., 1990.

Margen, Sheldon, and the Editors of the University of California at Berkeley Wellness Letter. *The Wellness Encyclopedia of Food and Nutrition.* New York: Health Letter Associates, 1992.

Morgan, Dr. Brian L. *Nutrition Prescription.* New York: Crown Publishers, 1987.

Ornish, Dean. *Eat More, Weigh Less.* New York: HarperCollins, 1993.

Winter, Ruth. *A Consumer's Guide to Medicines in Food.* New York: Crown Trade Paperbacks, 1995.

Index

Index

Cheese
  alternatives to, 48
  mozzarella, 153, 163
  power of, 183
  serving measurement, 169
  in weight-loss plan, 163
Cherries
  power of, 30, 42
  recipe, Baked Apples with Cherries and
      Walnuts, 333
  serving measurement, 165
Chestnuts, 37, 129, 131, 138
Chicken
  breast, 36
  power of, 149–50, 184
  marinated, 232–33
  serving measurement, 168
  in weight-loss plan, 162–63
Chick-peas, 115, 117–18, 177, 211
Chicory, 73–74
  serving measurement, 166
Chili
  powder, 214
  recipe, Vegetable Chili, 285
  sauce, 304
Chinese mushroom, 79
Chinese stir-fry, 77, 79
Chives
  power of, 19, 27–28, 92–94
  recipe, Mustard Chive Pasta Sauce, 307
Chloride, 10
Chlorogenic acid, 18
Cholesterol, see Cholesterol level, dietary
      influences
  diet and, 174
  types of, 21
Cholesterol level, dietary influences
  alliums, 94
  diet and, 174
  fruits and, 44
  garlic and, 93
  legumes and, 115
  mushrooms and, 80
  nuts and, 133, 139
  oat bran and, 104
  seeds and, 133
  soy and, 123
  whole grains and, 140
Chromium, sources of, 140
Chronic fatigue, 24
Chutney
  Cranberry, 297
  Pineapple Apricot, 298
Cilantro, recipes with, 207, 267, 271, 279–80, 289,
      294–95
Cinnamon, recipes with, 217–18, 244, 249–50,
      297, 310–11, 313, 318–19, 323–25,
      331–32, 338–39, 342–43, 347–51, 354
Citrus, 22–23, 26, 28
Citrus Asparagus Salad, 152
Citrus fruit, 19, 42, 44, 150, 174
Clams, 36, 168, 177
Cloves
  power of, 97
  recipes with, 214, 243, 297, 313, 318
Coconut oil, 183

Coconuts, 130, 136, 346
Coffee, 97
Collagen, dietary influences on, 20, 23, 25–26, 45
Collards
  power of, 30, 68, 71, 178–79
  serving measurement, 166
Colon cancer, 16, 18, 24, 27, 65, 69, 86, 89, 92,
      106
Concord grapes, 51
Condiments, 36–37
Constipation, 24, 87, 106
Copper, sources of, 133, 140–41
Corn
  power of, 23, 101, 103, 109–10
  recipes, 268, 289, 317
Corn bread, serving measurement, 167
Cornish hen, serving measurement, 168
Cornmeal, 110
Corn on the cob, serving measurement, 167
Coronary heart disease, 21
Cottage cheese, 169, 184
Coumarins, sources of, 13, 28, 106–7, 114, 123,
      140
Couscous
  power of, 35, 102, 109
  recipes
    Basil Couscous with Squash, 274
    Couscous Dinner Salad, 154
    Fruited Couscous Salad, 233
    Lemon-zested Couscous Dinner Salad, 234
Crab, 36, 168
Crackers, 35, 167, 176
Cranberries
  Apple Cranberry Crisp, 331
  Cranberry Chutney, 155
Cream/cream sauces, 183
Cream of Mushroom Soup, 212
Crenshaws, 49–50
Crockpots, 118
Cruciferous vegetables
  buying and preparation guidelines, 70–71
  cancer and, 179
  defined, 67
  phytochemicals in, 140
  power of, 15, 17–19, 25–28, 68–69, 140
  types of, 67–68, 71–73
  in weight-loss plan, 162
Cucumbers
  power of, 28, 174, 184
  recipes
    Cucumber Salad, 153–54
    Warm Salad, 229
  serving measurement, 165
Cumin, 214, 285
Curry Sauce, 154

Daidzein, 28, 123
Daikon, 184, 264
Daily calorie intake, 160–62
Dairy foods/products
  daily calorie intake servings, 163, 168–69
  osteoporosis and, 178–79
  power of, 31
  in weight-loss plan, 163
Dandelion greens, 74
Dates, 165, 322

Genistein, 19, 28, 123
Ginger mayonnaise, 155, 163
    recipe, Grilled Tuna Steaks with Ginger
        Mayonnaise, 292
Glutathione-S-transferase, 19, 94
Glycogen, 8
Gouda cheese, 169
Grains
  as fiber sources, 151
  whole, *see* Whole grains
Granny Smith apples, 43
Granola, 108
Grape cure, 51
Grapefruit
  power of, 27, 151, 177
  serving measurement, 165
Grape-Nuts cereal, 323
Grape-Nuts Muffins, 154
Grapes
  power of, 19, 22–23, 26, 41–43, 46, 50–51,
      151, 177
  serving measurement, 165
Great Northern beans, 151
Greek Tabbouleh Salad, 153
Green bananas, 47
Green beans, 240
Green chiles, 37
Green grapes, 50–51
Green leafy vegetables
  buying and preparation guidelines, 70–71
  osteoporosis and, 178
  phytochemicals in, 140
  power of, 17, 22, 25, 30, 68–69, 140
  types of, 71–73
  in weight-loss plan, 162
Green pepper
  power of, 150
Greens
  power of, 150
Green tea, 28
Grits, serving measurement, 167
Ground chicken, 36
Ground turkey, 36

Halibut, Baked, with Herb Bread Crumb
    Topping, 288
Hazelnuts, 37, 129–30, 331
Head and neck cancers, 17
Health, diet and, 5–7, 20–21, 29
Heart attacks, 46, 93
Heart disease, *see* Cardiovascular disease; *specific*
    types of heart disease
  cholesterol and, 174
  dietary influences, 27
  fruits and, 140
  garlic and, 89, 174
  soy/soy products and, 141
  vegetables and, 140
  whole grains and, 106
Hemorrhoids, 24, 106
Herbs, *see also specific types of herbs*
  as pantry necessities, 37–38
  power of, 30
Herpes simplex virus, 46
Herring, 176
Hesperidin, 26, 45

Hickory nuts, 131
High-density lipoprotein (HDL), 21,
    175–76
High-fat foods, 31
Hijiki, 238
  recipe, Tossed Salad, 155
Honeydew, 165, 343
Horseradish, 68, 296
Hot chile peppers, 19, 23
Hot peppers, 28
Hubbard squash, 62
Hummus, 154, 207
Hydrogenated fats, 176
Hydrogenated vegetable oil, 183
Hypertension, 4, 10, 21–22, 177

Immune system
  general dietary influences, 7, 14, 22, 80
  mushrooms and, 140
  nuts and, 141
  sea vegetables and, 86
  seeds and, 141
Indigestion, 87
Indol–3-carbinol, 19
Indoles, sources of, 13, 26, 69, 114, 140
Infection, and dietary influences, 4, 21–22
Injera, 105
Iodine, sources of, 86, 140
Iron, sources of, 44, 73, 86, 93, 133, 139–40,
    150
Irritable bowel, 24
Isoflavones, 25, 29, 141
Isothiocyanates, 13, 19, 27, 140

Jalapeño pepper, 37, 285, 294
Jam, preparation guidelines, 48
Japanese diet, 19, 122
Jarlsberg cheese, 169
Jelly, preparation guidelines, 37, 48
Jicama, 184
Juice
  apple, 233, 291, 297, 298, 302, 313, 347,
    350
  lemon, 207, 223–24, 226–28, 234, 237, 240,
    252, 256, 289, 297, 300, 304, 313, 320,
    333–34, 338, 343–44
  lime, 206, 218, 223, 267, 279, 289, 291, 294,
    301, 338–39
  orange, 150, 179, 248, 299, 301–2, 304,
    310–11, 332, 334, 353
  pineapple, 204, 218, 290, 301, 346
  power of, 34–35
  V–8, 215
Juniper berries, 251

Kale
  power of, 18, 26, 30, 68, 71–72, 149–50, 174,
    178–79
  recipes
    Bulgur, Kale, and Carrot Pilaf, 277
    Kale Soup, 72, 153, 211
  serving measurement, 166
Kanten, 85
  Blackberry, 153–54, 347
Kasha, 35, 184
Ketchup, 37

Index

Index